Color Atlas of

VENOUS DISEASE

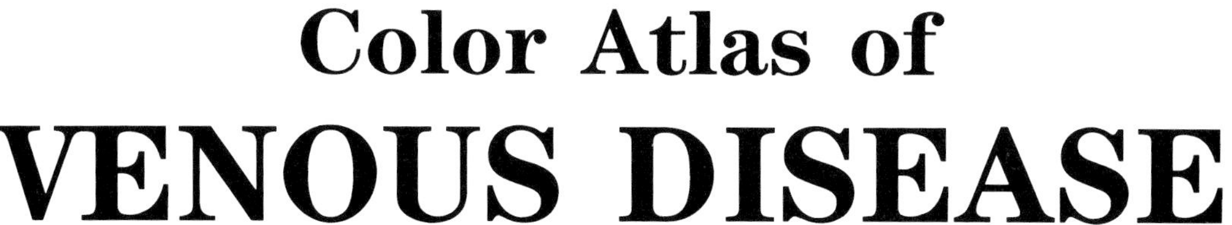

Color Atlas of VENOUS DISEASE

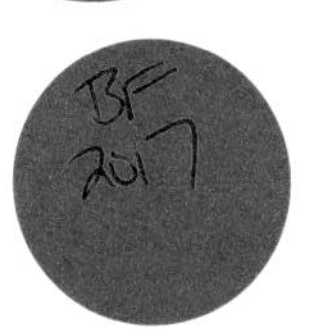

Henner Altenkämper
Evangelical Hospital, Plettenburg, Germany
President, German Phlebological Society

Matthias Eldenburg
Phlebologist
Düsseldorf, Germany

with contributions from

Franz Platz
Academic Director, Department of Anatomy
University of Freiburg, Germany

Reinhard Poche
Professor, Department of Pathology
University of Bielefeld, Germany

and a Foreword by
Jochen Staubesand
Professor Emeritus, Department of Anatomy
University of Freiburg, Germany

English edition translated and edited by
Walter P. de Groot, MD, FACS
Swedish Medical Center, Seattle, USA
Past President, North American Society of Phlebology

and a Foreword by
Ivor G. Schraibman, MCh, FRCS(Ed), FRCS
Consultant Surgeon, Birch Hill Hospital, Rochdale, UK
Steering Committee Member, Venous Forum, Royal Society of Medicine

J. B. Lippincott Company
Philadelphia

Acknowledgements

Illustrations have been reproduced by kind permission of the following:

1–10: from J. Staubesand (editor): Sobotta – Atlas of Human Anatomy, Volume 2, Nineteenth impression, Urban & Schwarzenberg, Munich – Vienna – Baltimore, 1988.
11–19: Franz Platz, Freiburg.
20/21: from W. Hach Die Primäre Varikose.
22–25, 26, 27, 29, 34–37, 39–41, 46–55, 57–78, 82–86, 90–124: Henner Altenkämper, Plettenberg.
25, 28, 30–33, 38, 42–45, 56, 79–81, 87–89: Horst Gerlach, Mannheim.
32 Duplex scan: Pauline Raymond-Martimbeau, Dallas.
125–139 Reinhard Poche, Bielefeld.

Published by Manson Publishing Ltd., 1994 from the German edition published by Schlütersche Verlagsanstalt und Druckerei GmbH & Co.
ISBN: 1-874545-01-4

A CIP catalogue record for this book is available from the British Library.

Copublished and distributed in North America by J.B. Lippincott Company, Philadelphia, 1994.
ISBN: 0-397-51395-X
Library of Congress Cataloging in Publication Data applied for.

Typeset by Setrite Typesetters Ltd., Hong Kong.
Printed and bound by Schlütersche Verlagsanstalt und Druckerei GmbH & Co.

Contents

Foreword (*Jochen Staubesand*) 7

Foreword to the English language edition (*Ivor Schraibman*) 7

Preface 8

Translator and editor's note to the English language edition
(*Walter P. de Groot*) 8

Introduction:
The clinical importance of venous disorders 9
Henner Altenkämper/Matthias Eldenburg

1. Anatomy of the venous and arterial systems of the lower limb 12
Jochen Staubesand/Franz Platz

2. Phlebological conditions 28
Henner Altenkämper/Matthias Eldenburg
Types of varicose veins 28
Chronic venous insufficiency 58
Inflammatory conditions of the veins 62
Venous ulceration 73
Angiodysplasias 82
Oedema. 83

3. Histopathology of the leg veins with special reference to phlebosclerosis 91
Reinhard Poche

Select bibliography 110

Index. 111

Foreword

Growing interest in diseases of the veins is reflected in, among other things, the increasing number of textbooks and reference works on phlebology. Until now, however, an atlas such as this by Dr Altenkämper and Dr Eldenburg, has not appeared in the literature.
Using predominantly photographs to illustrate conditions, the two authors have succeeded in producing an excellent survey covering the diverse problems of venous disease.
They begin by depicting the anatomical and pathophysiological bases of venous conditions and go on to describe physical and up-to-date imaging methods of clinical examination.
Outstanding photographs and radiographs, supplemented by phlebograms, demonstrate the variety of diseases affecting leg veins. A survey of therapeutic methods is followed by one of Reinhard Poche's introductory sequences of histopathological sections, with special emphasis on phlebosclerosis – pictures of great aesthetic appeal and didactic value. Such illustrations have not been published before in this number and variety.
The excellent production quality of the book and the predominantly large illustrations make the subject easily accessible to the reader. I hope that *A Colour Atlas of Venous Disease* will achieve wide circulation. It opens the door to a group of diseases whose clinical, economic and health-policy significance is still underestimated by many. It arouses interest in the field of varicosis and thereby helps to serve the welfare of affected patients.

J. Staubesand, MD, Professor Emeritus
Formerly Director of the Institute of Anatomy at the Albert-Ludwigs University, Freiburg, Germany

Foreword to the English language edition

Medicine in the English-speaking countries has traditionally lagged behind Continental Europe in the study of phlebology and the provision of phlebological services. Venous disease has usually fallen within the remit of the general surgeon because it seems to combine a lack of excitement (no dramatic operations) with a potentially threatening work-load. Perhaps because of a better doctor/patient numerical ratio, phlebology in Continental Europe developed into a discipline of its own, only peripherally overlapping surgery.
This changed with the inauguration of the Venous Forum of the Royal Society of Medicine in London in 1983, and, more recently, with the establishment of the American Venous Forum and the North American Society of Phlebology. There has been a burgeoning of research and treatment of venous disease in Britain and the USA, to the extent that phlebology is no longer considered a Cinderella backwater. This enthusiasm has in turn been communicated to phlebologist colleagues on the Continent, with an increase of interest and quality of work in venous thrombosis, ulcus cruris and varicose veins, augmented by the need to be cost-effective, particularly so in the treatment of varicose veins. Rising patient expectations in a field affecting 10% of the adult population could swamp hard-pressed health services and draw resources from other areas of health care. The answer lies in increased efficiency – day case surgery, leg ulcer clinics and audit – to point the way to higher standards with less complications and more efficient throughput.
This book is timely and commends itself to all phlebologists and to a wide range of physicians, surgeons and other health professionals interested in venous disease. Doctors Altenkämper and Eldenburg have made us privy to their vast clinical experience and provided a detailed guide describing the indications for and usefulness of sophisticated investigative techniques, with many beautifully clear and precise illustrations. With this sort of Bible in hand, we should be proselytizing our colleagues, showing them that phlebology is a discrete (though not narrow or exclusive) discipline which can be practised by anyone with the requisite enthusiasm and knowledge.

Ivor Schraibman, MCh, FRCS(Ed), FRCS
Birch Hill Hospital, Rochdale

Preface

The needs of an extremely large number of patients suffering from phlebological conditions are increasingly being met by a medical profession that is beginning to examine venous ailments in practical and efficient ways.
The aim of this book is to represent venous anatomy, venous physiological correlations and phlebological disease in a clear and clinically relevant way. We therefore chose to represent the subject by means of an atlas.
We have started with anatomy, using remarkable drawings and photographs, for which we are grateful to Dr Jochen Staubesand and to Dr Franz Platz. We then give some insight into important areas of diagnosis and differential diagnosis using physical examination and imaging techniques. We are particularly grateful to our colleague Dr Horst Gerlach for his excellent photographs of phlebological conditions.
We would also like to make mention of Dr Reinhard Poche's contribution, covering the histopathology of the veins with special reference to phlebosclerosis, and probably published here for the first time in atlas form.
Finally, the thanks of the authors and other physicians are due to our publishers who, by issuing this book, have contributed to the educational process in phlebology.

The Authors

Translator and editor's note to the English language edition

The enthusiasm for the study and treatment of venous disorders has spread from Continental Europe and Great Britain to the United States over the past decade.
Subjects such as deep vein thrombosis and surgery of the deep veins have always been well represented in the United States, with leading innovations such as the DeWeese and Greenfield vena cava filtres for the prevention of pulmonary embolism and the De Palma bypass operation for deep vein obstruction. Although these subjects are certainly also studied in the new phlebology, its main interest and its innovations are in the field of superficial venous disorders, a subject which so far tended to be neglected, possibly because it was, wrongly, considered not to be dramatic enough.
This *Colour Atlas of Venous Disease* is not meant to be a textbook of phlebology. Complicated diagnostic procedures and treatment methods are only briefly alluded to. Rather, it shows, as its name implies, all the visual aspects of the natural history of superficial venous disorders. As such, this book is unique in the present literature.
Chapter 1 deals with the anatomy of the superficial venous system. The purely Latin nomenclature of the original German edition has been translated into the anglicized terms customary in the Anglo-American literature, except for a few terms used in special anatomical dissections (e.g. "ramus fibularis" in Figure 17).
Chapter 2 offers a rich display of clinical presentations of varicose vein disease in its various stages. It will create in the reader a familiarity with clinical presentations which normally can only be built up through several years of clinical practice.
Chapter 3 shows the microscopic imagery of varicose vein disease. The author uses a terminology with a sense of detail and sophistication which will be a pleasant and enriching surprise to many.
All in all, a beautiful atlas of varicose vein disease, which will be a pleasant and useful companion in the exploration of the fascinating new field of phlebology.

Walter P. de Groot, MD, FACS
Seattle, USA

Introduction: The clinical importance of venous disorders

Henner Altenkämper/Matthias Eldenburg

The frequency and clinical significance of venous disorders are often underestimated. As early as the 1930s, peripheral venous disorders were shown to be the third most common condition in the Health Survey Study, a study of chronic disorders in the English speaking countries and Denmark.
The Tübingen study, covering what was then West Germany, showed that 24 million people between the ages of 20 and 70 had changes in their venous walls. Twelve million of these showed signs of main trunk varicosis, 5.3 million suffered from chronic venous insufficiency, and 1.3 million patients had a varicose ulcer or a past history of ulcers.
In our opinion, 50% of women and 25% of men have a venous condition. It is reasonable to extrapolate that every second patient in a doctor's waiting room is also a vein patient. In view of these statistics, it is hard to explain why the medical world is so ineffective and shows so little concern about such a widespread disease.
Usually, only acute venous disorders, such as superficial thrombophlebitis or acute deep vein thrombosis, receive attention and are properly diagnosed and treated. For example, a varicose ulcer, as part of a post-thrombotic syndrome, can lead to disability of the patient and often only then causes the patient to be treated properly.
The prevention of serious venous disorders is the neglected stepchild of our medical health care systems: can many of the richest countries in the world, despite their other impressive medical accomplishments, afford to ignore this worldwide disease, especially with the increasing number of people whose occupations require prolonged standing and sitting?
The recognition of phlebological disorders and their adequate basic treatment, as well as interaction with a vein specialist where needed, should become routine for every doctor.
Even when the patient does not consult a physician primarily concerning a venous condition, history taking and clinical examination should look for evidence of venous disease to prevent possible complications and later damage. History taking should include questions about a feeling of heaviness in the legs, unexplained leg swelling, paresthesias, pain, leg cramps, possible past superficial phlebitis or thrombophlebitis, and pulmonary emboli. If the patient's answers suggest venous disease, a more specific inquiry should be made.
Information about the duration of symptoms and past treatment are of clinical importance. Also important are risk factors such as medication intake, family history of venous disease, pregnancies, occupations which require prolonged standing or sitting, obesity, sports activities and many other factors. All these data are recorded in a phlebological chart as shown (Diagram A).
This is followed by clinical venous examination, the findings of which are documented in an examination chart (Diagram B). History taking and clinical examination can, and should be, done by every primary care physician. If a unidirectional or bidirectional Doppler is available, a first examination can provide valuable information about the nature and extent of a venous disorder which presents itself. Light-reflection rheography (LRR), venous occlusion plethysmography, venous pressure measurements, venography or duplex examination can be done by a phlebologist, and these studies will enable him to recommend the best treatment. This treatment can consist of compression, sclerotherapy, or surgery.

A

Phlebological history

Name: ______ Date of birth ______ Date: ______

General history: ______

Phlebological history ______
Onset of symptoms ______
Leg swelling ______
Heaviness ______
Nocturnal calf cramps ______
Pruritus ______

Thrombophlebitis Yes/No

Deep vein thrombosis Yes/No

Risk profile: ______
Heredity ______
Standing occupation ______
Contracept./oestrogen Rx ______
Weight ______
Number of pregnancies ______

Previous treatment:
Sclerotherapy ______
Compression ______
Surgery ______
Medications ______
Other ______

Suggested treatment: ______

B

Perforators

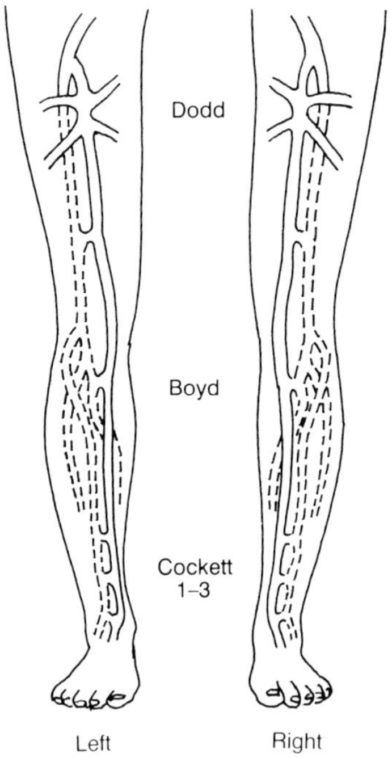

Venous status

Status	Upper leg R	Upper leg L	Lower leg R	Lower leg L	Foot R	Foot L
Oedema/lymphoedema						
Stasis dermatitis						
Hyperpigmentation						
Atrophie blanche						
Venous ulcer						
Corona phlebectatica						
Thrombophlebitis						

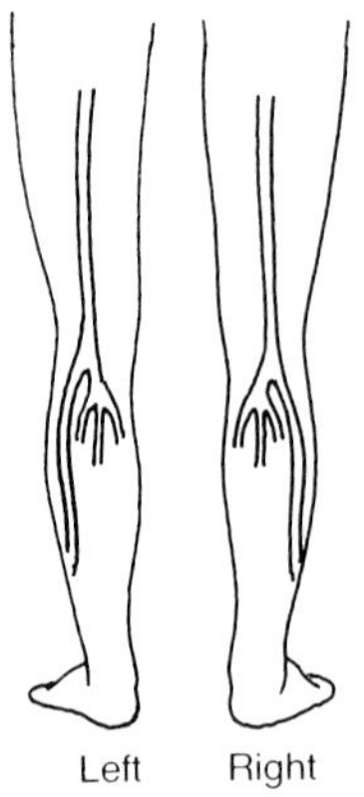

Doppler	R	L
Resp. fluct./fem.		
LSV reflux (junction)		
Resp. fluct./popl.		
SSV reflux		
Art. pressure (mmHg)	**R**	**L**
Post. tib. art.		
Brachial art.		
LRR/PPG	**R**	**L**
Refilling time		
Refilling time with tourn.		

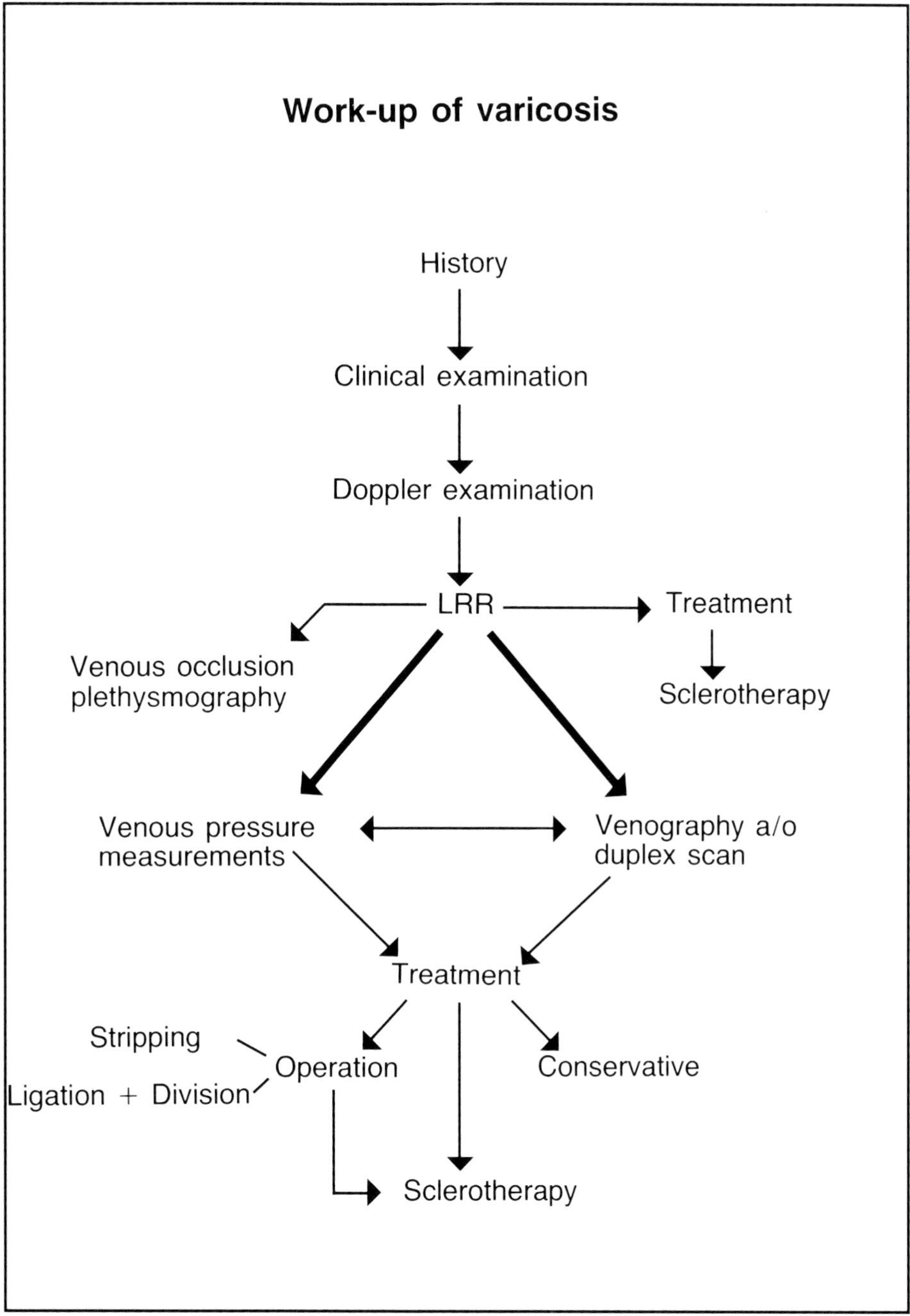
Work-up of varicosis
History
Clinical examination
Doppler examination
LRR
Treatment
Sclerotherapy
Venous occlusion plethysmography
Venous pressure measurements
Venography a/o duplex scan
Treatment
Stripping
Operation
Ligation + Division
Conservative
Sclerotherapy

1. Anatomy of the venous and arterial systems of the lower limb

Franz Platz/Jochen Staubesand

1

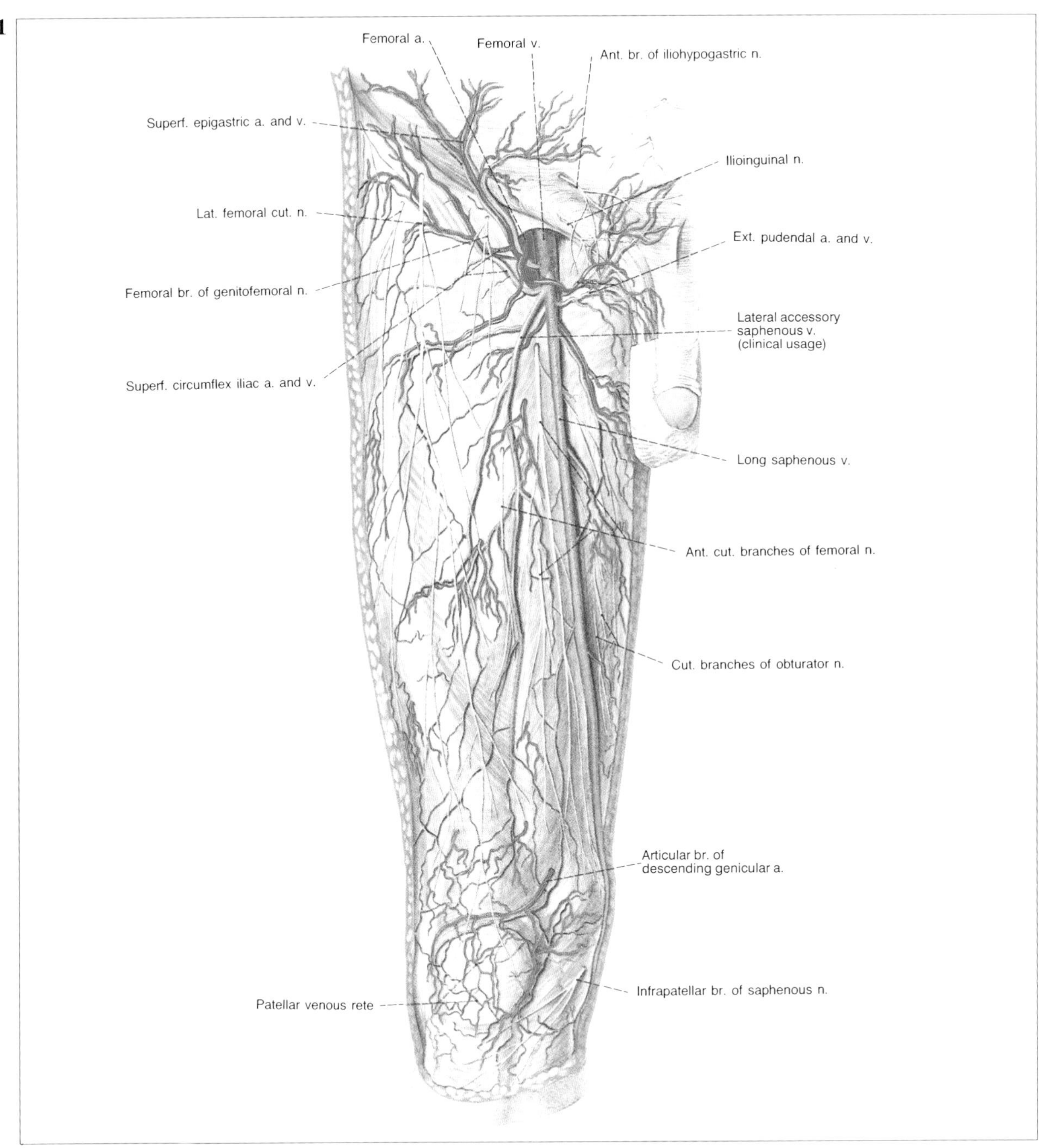

1: Superficial veins, arteries and cutaneous nerves of the anterior aspect of the right thigh.

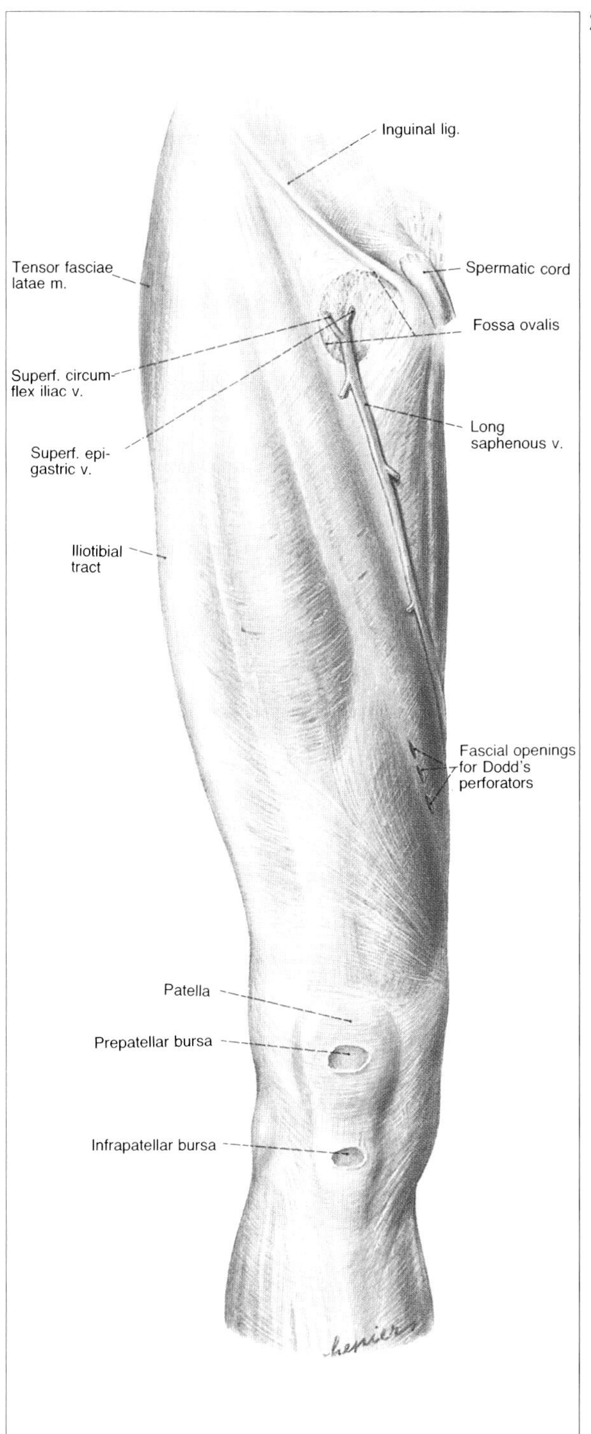

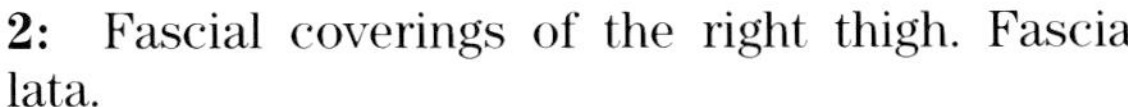

2: Fascial coverings of the right thigh. Fascia lata.

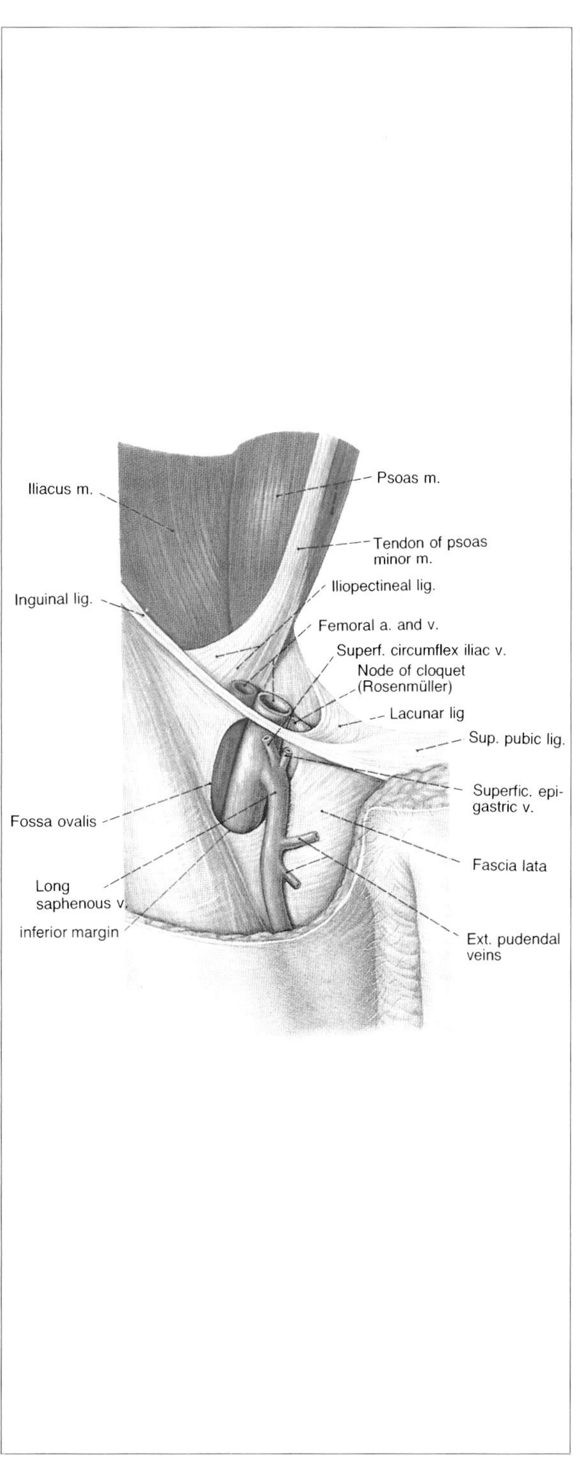

3: Fossa ovalis and main structures of the vascular lacuna.

4

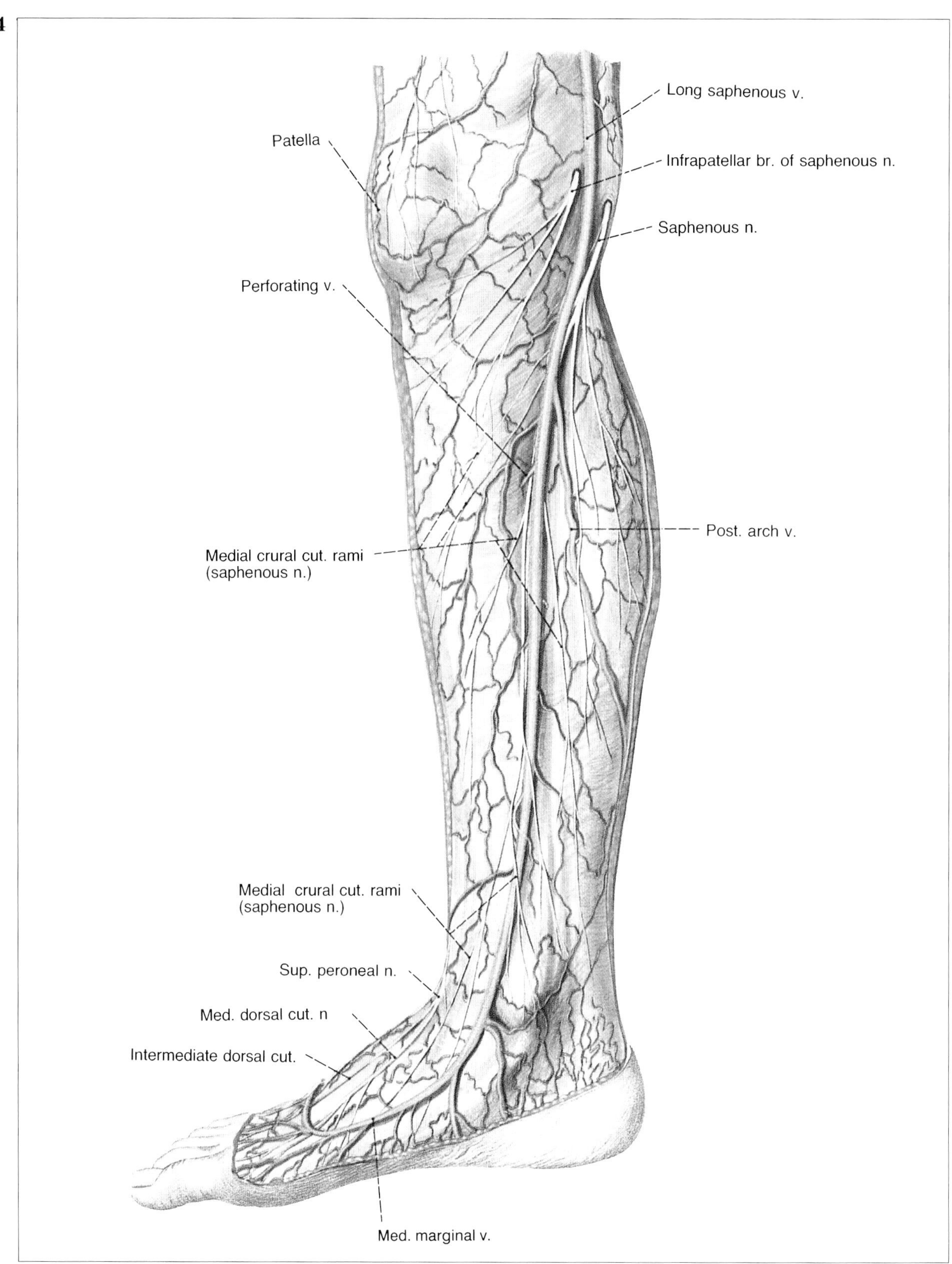

4: Superficial veins and cutaneous nerves of the right lower leg and foot. Medial aspect.

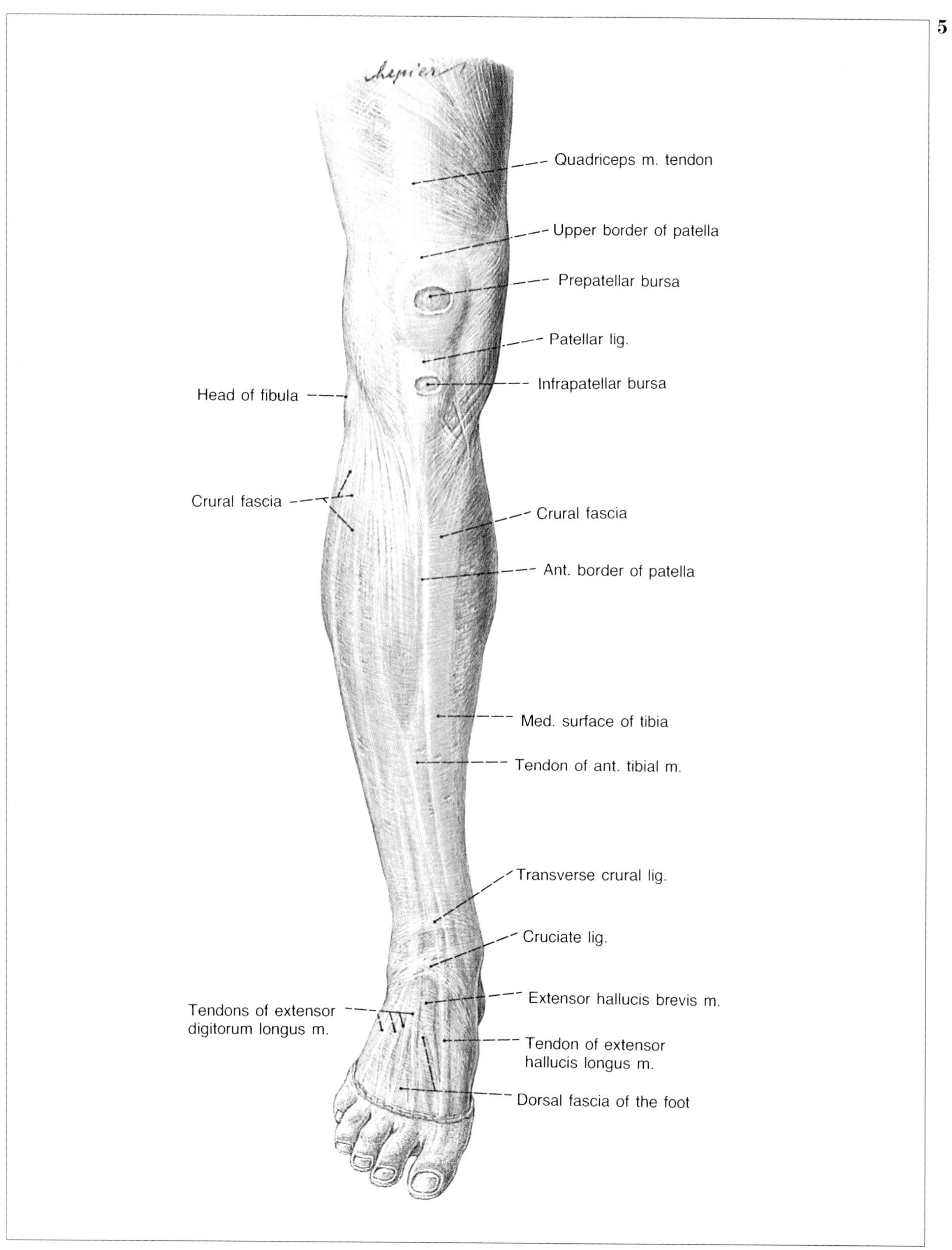

5: Crural fascia of the lower leg and dorsal fascia of the foot.

6

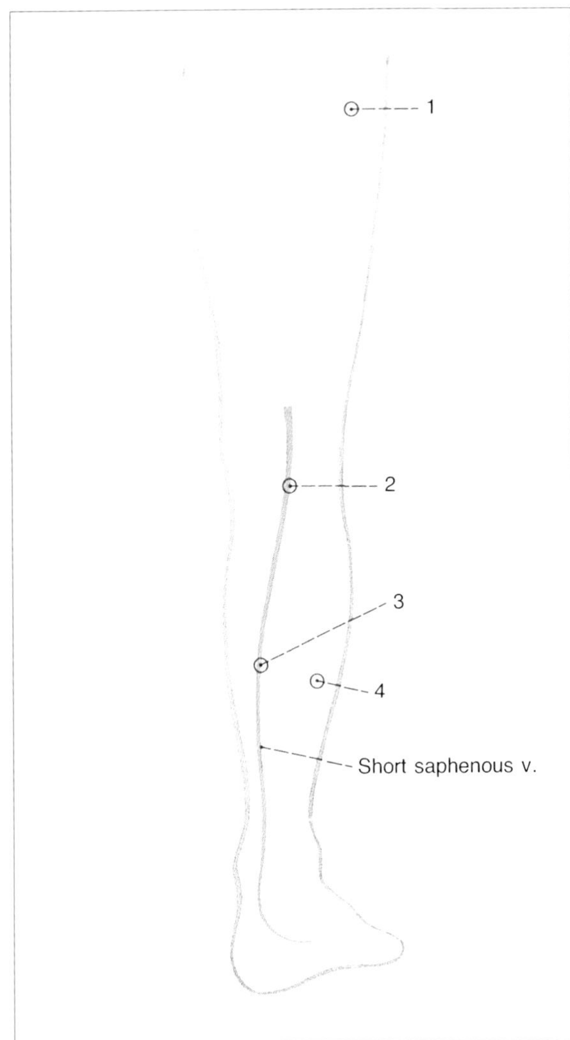

6: Clinically important perforating veins on the dorsal aspect of the leg.

1 = profunda perforator (Hach)
2 = popliteal fossa perforator
3 = May's vein
4 = lateral perforator

7

1
2
Long saphenous v.
3
4
5
6

7: Clinically important perforating veins on the medial aspect of the leg (Hach 1986).

1 = Dodd's veins
2 = Hunter's vein
3 = Boyd's vein
4 = post. arch vein
5 = Sherman's vein
6 = Cockett's veins

8

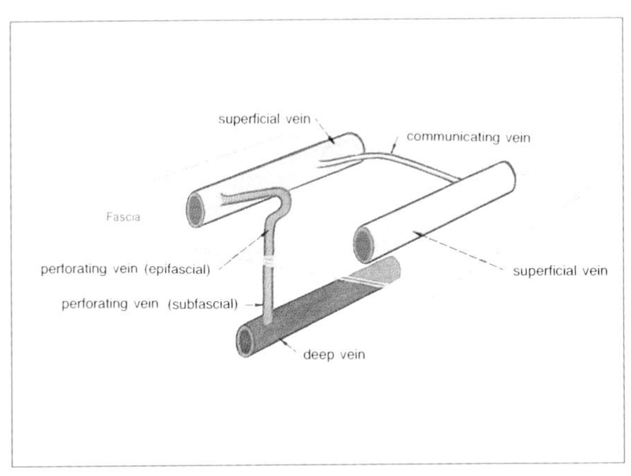

8: Schematic representation of the triple vein system of the lower limbs.

superficial veins = light blue
deep veins = dark blue
perforating veins = medium blue
fascia = grey

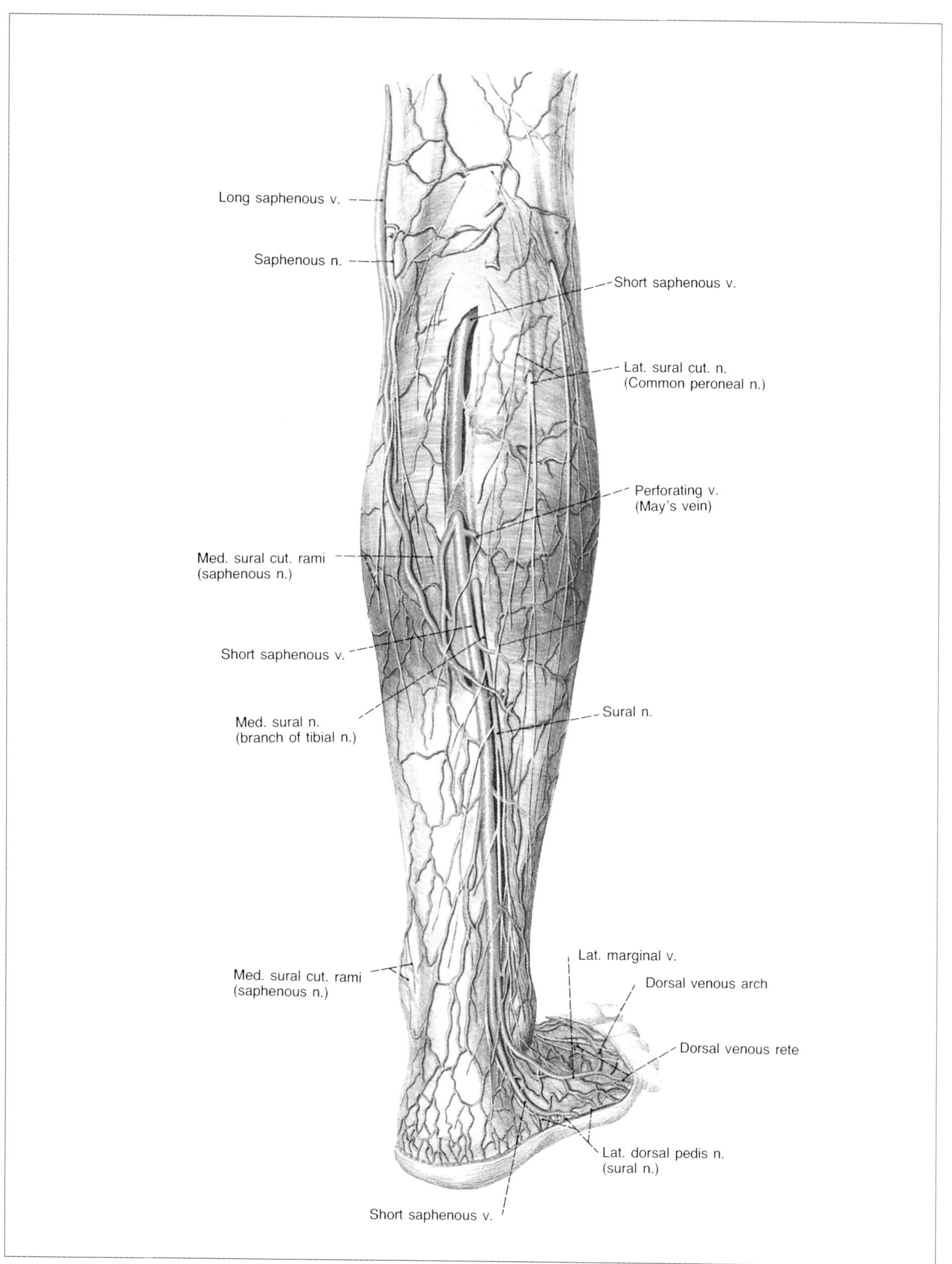

9: Superficial veins and cutaneous nerves of right lower leg and foot. Dorsal aspect.

10

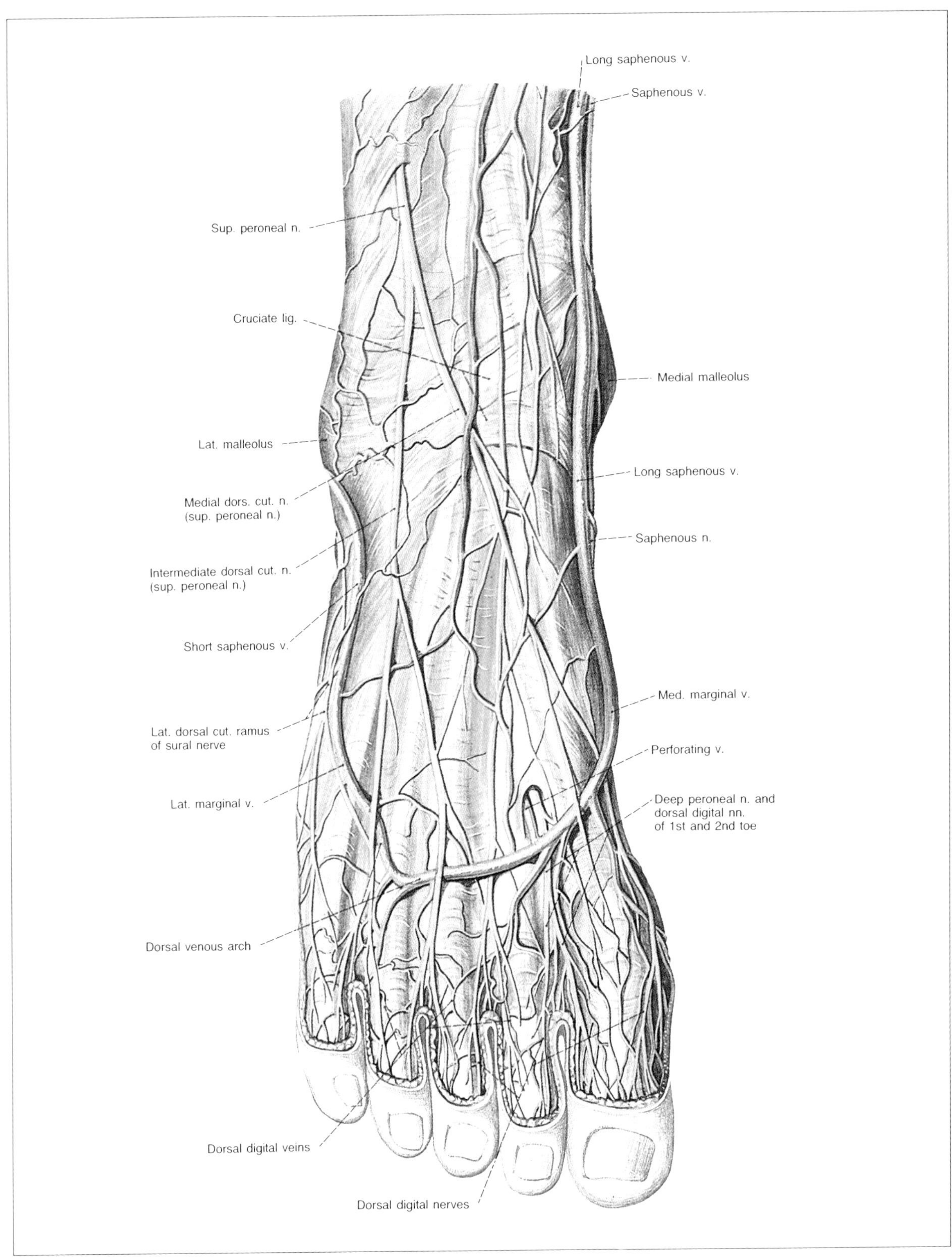

10: Epifascial veins and cutaneous nerves of the right foot.

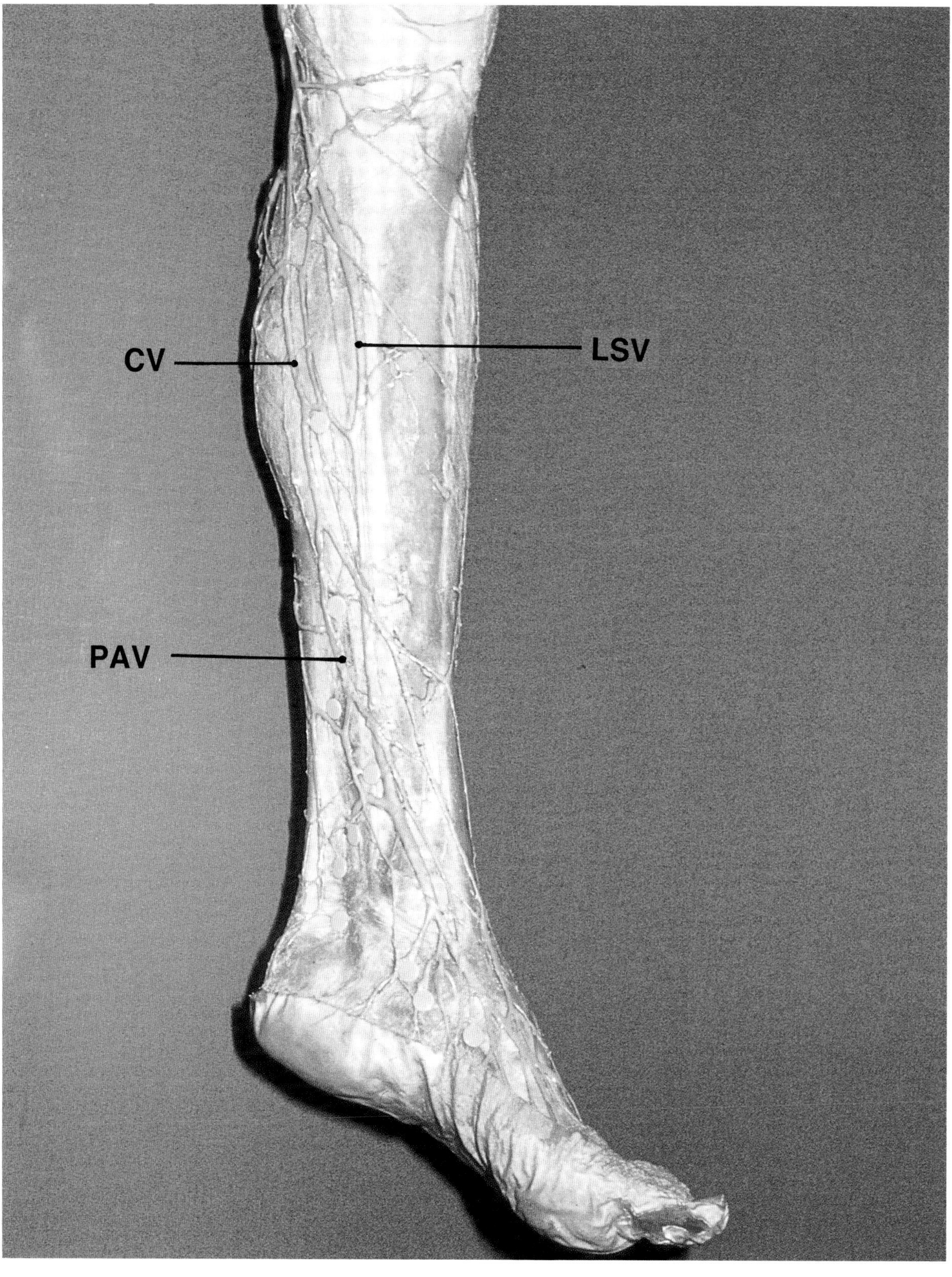

11: Left lower medial leg and foot with long saphenous vein (LSV), posterior arch vein (PAV) with irregular course, and communicating veins (CV). Fascial entrance points of perforating veins indicated in yellow. (Orig. Prep. by DR. F. PLATZ, Anat. Instit., Freiburg)

12

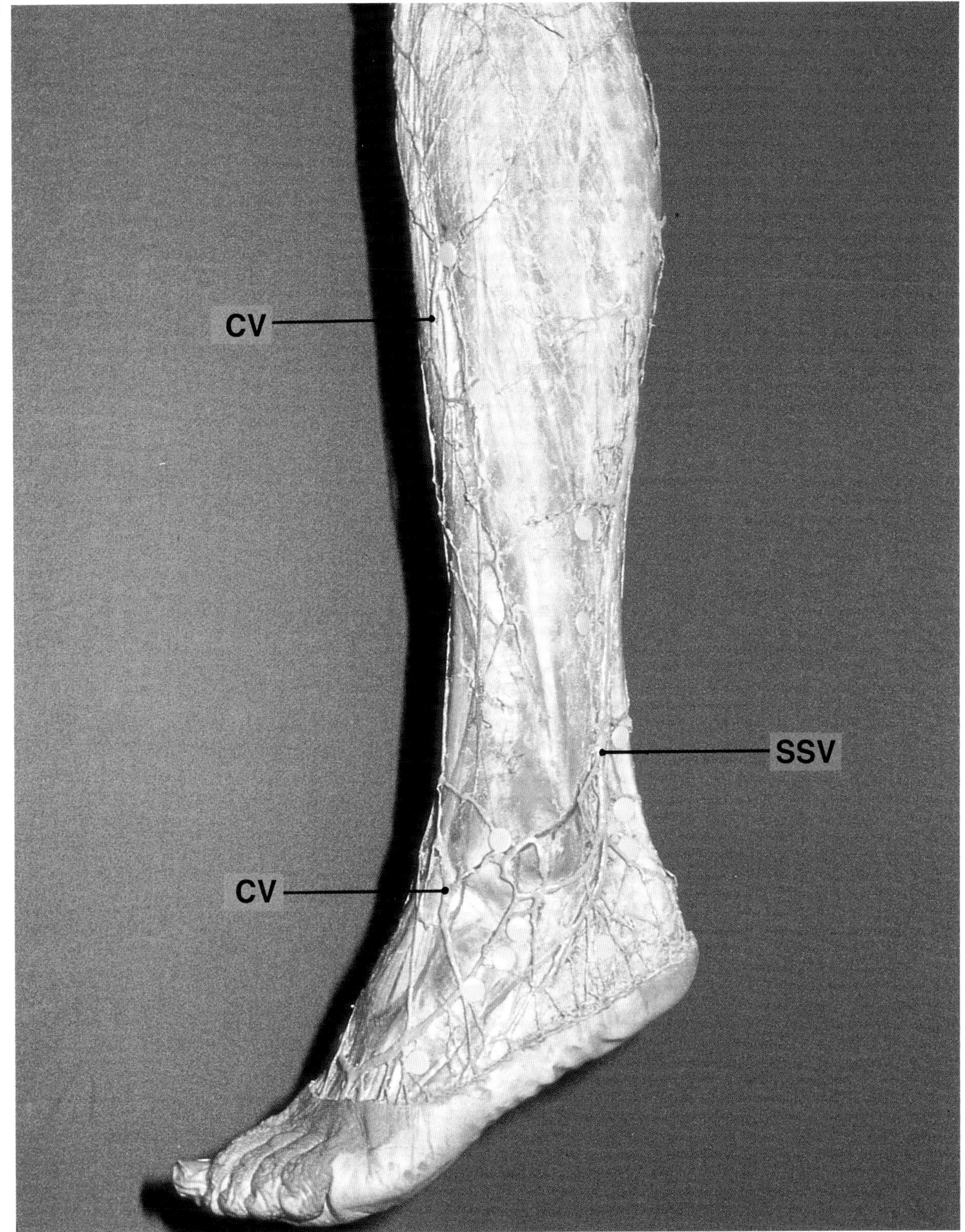

12: Left lower lateral leg with distal segment of short saphenous vein (SSV), communicating veins (CV) and entrance points of perforating veins (indicated in yellow). (Orig. Prep. by Dr. F. Platz, Anat. Instit., Freiburg)

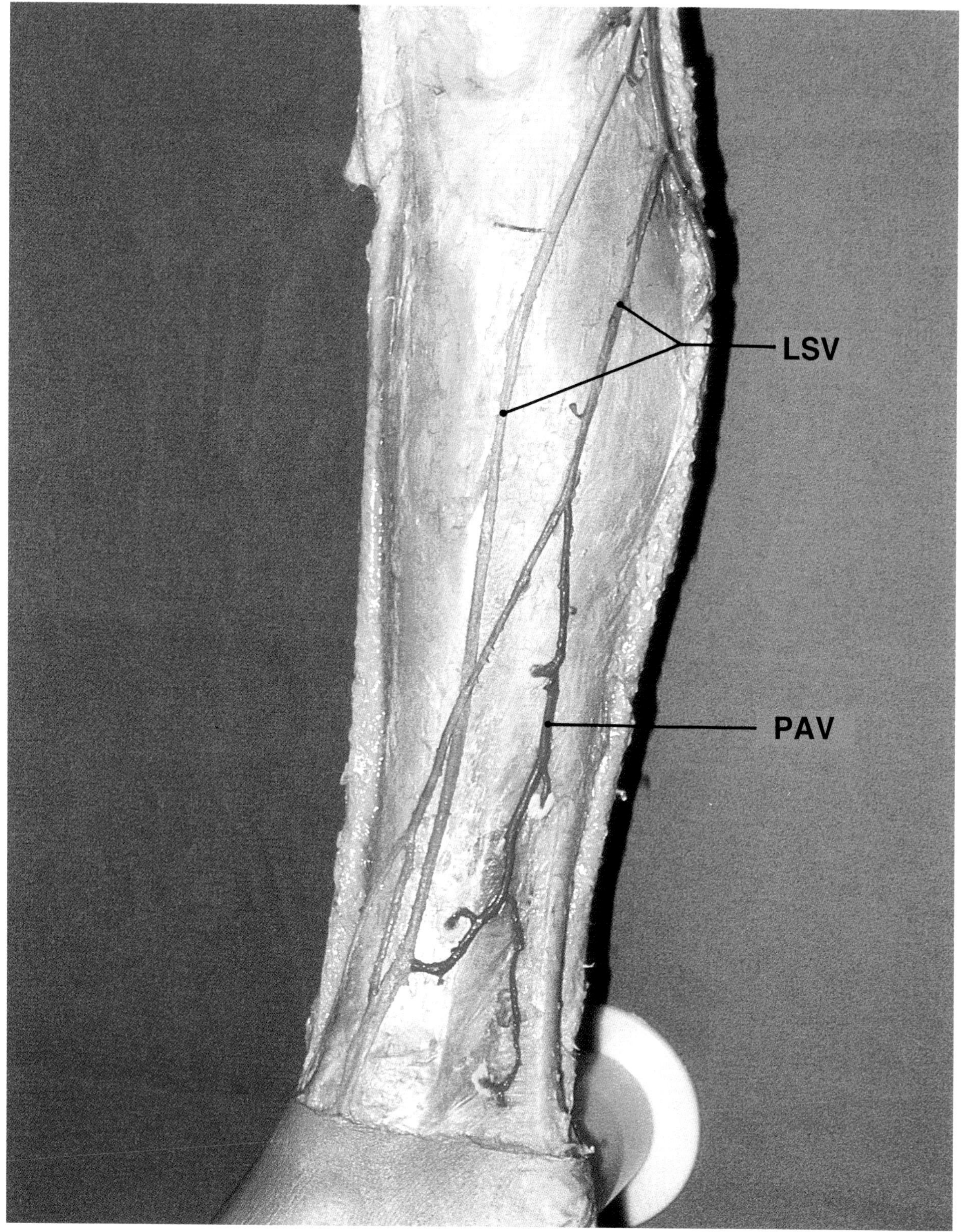

13: Right lower medial leg with double long saphenous vein (LSV). The posterior arch vein (PAV) connects the anterior and the posterior trunk. The perforating veins of the posterior arch vein are indicated in yellow. (Orig. Prep. by DR. G. ADELMANN and DR. F. PLATZ, Anat. Instit., Freiburg)

14

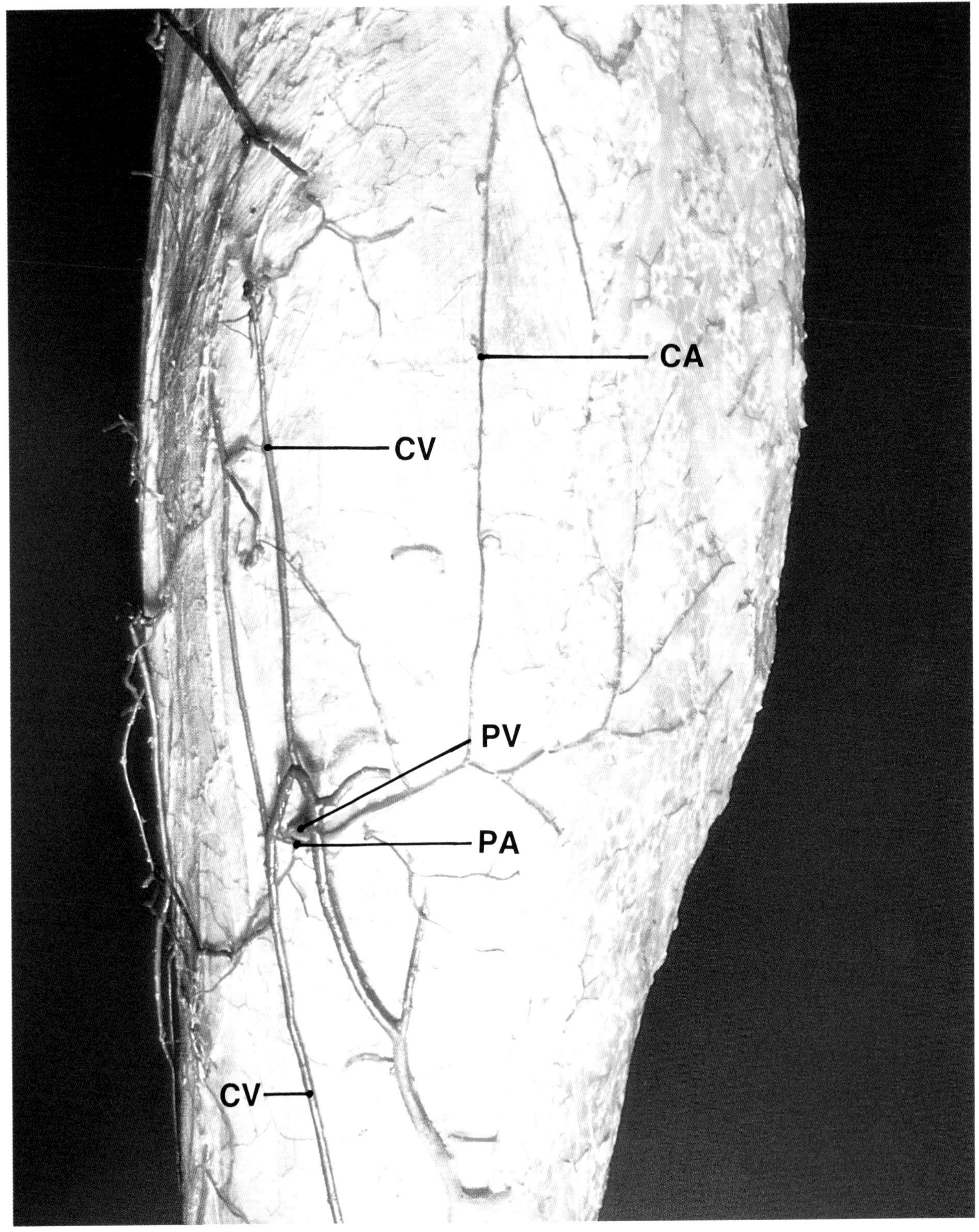

14: Posterolateral aspect of left calf. Perforating artery and vein (PA, PV) in fascial opening, anastomosing communicating veins (CV), and communicating artery (CA). The arterial (red) and venous (blue) vessels have been injected with liquid silicone rubber. (Orig. Prep. by DR. R. BAUMANN and DR. F. PLATZ, Anat. Instit., Freiburg)

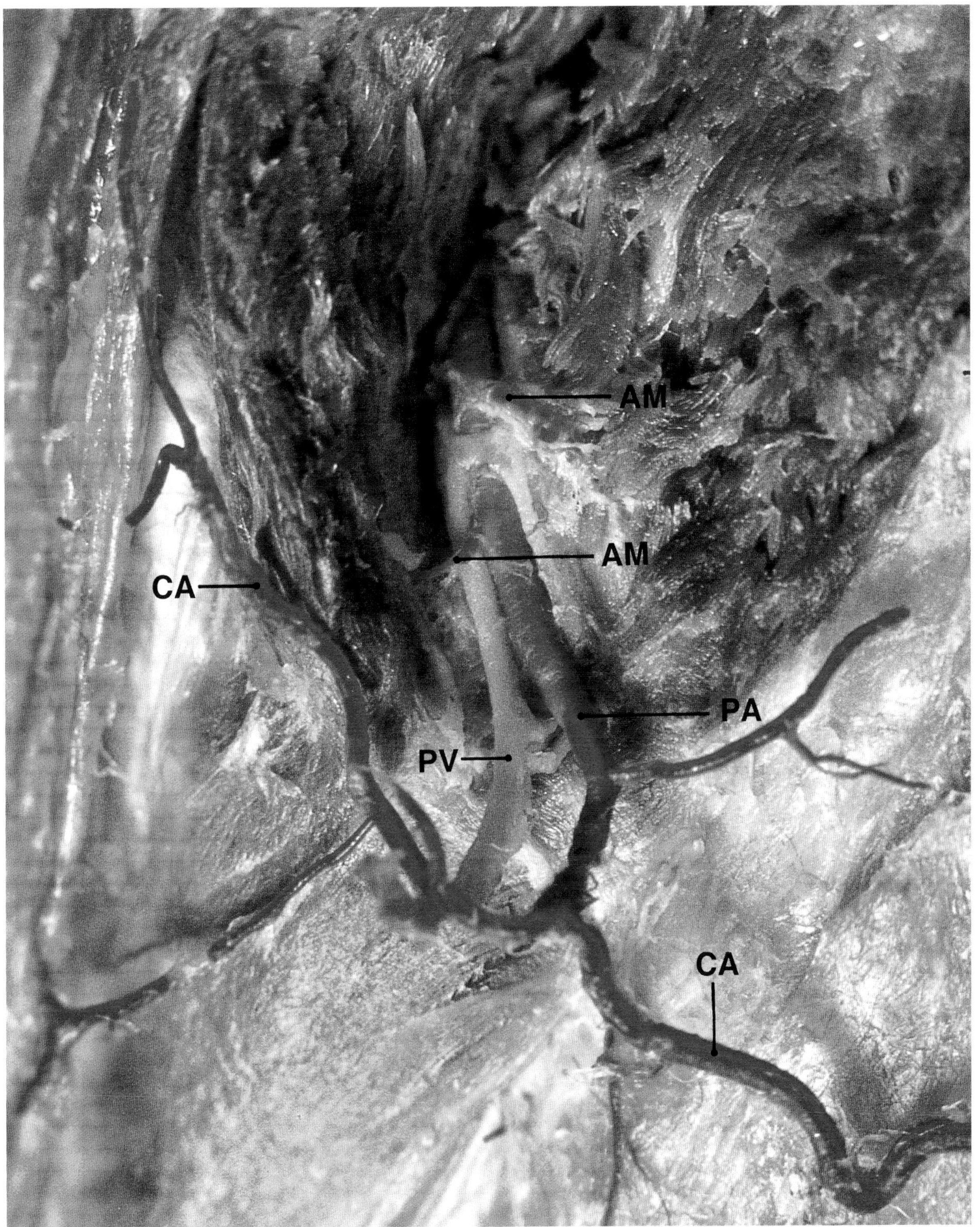

15: Dissected perforating artery and vein (PA, PV) at the lateral edge of the soleus muscle of the right lower leg, 21.5 cm proximal to the lateral malleolus. Take off from the fibular (peroneal) artery. Epifascial branchings of the communicating arteries (CA). Subfascial branches of the perforating artery to the musculature (AM). Arterial vascular bed injected with red silicone rubber. (Orig. Prep. by Dr. R. Baumann and Dr. F. Platz, Anat. Instit., Freiburg)

16

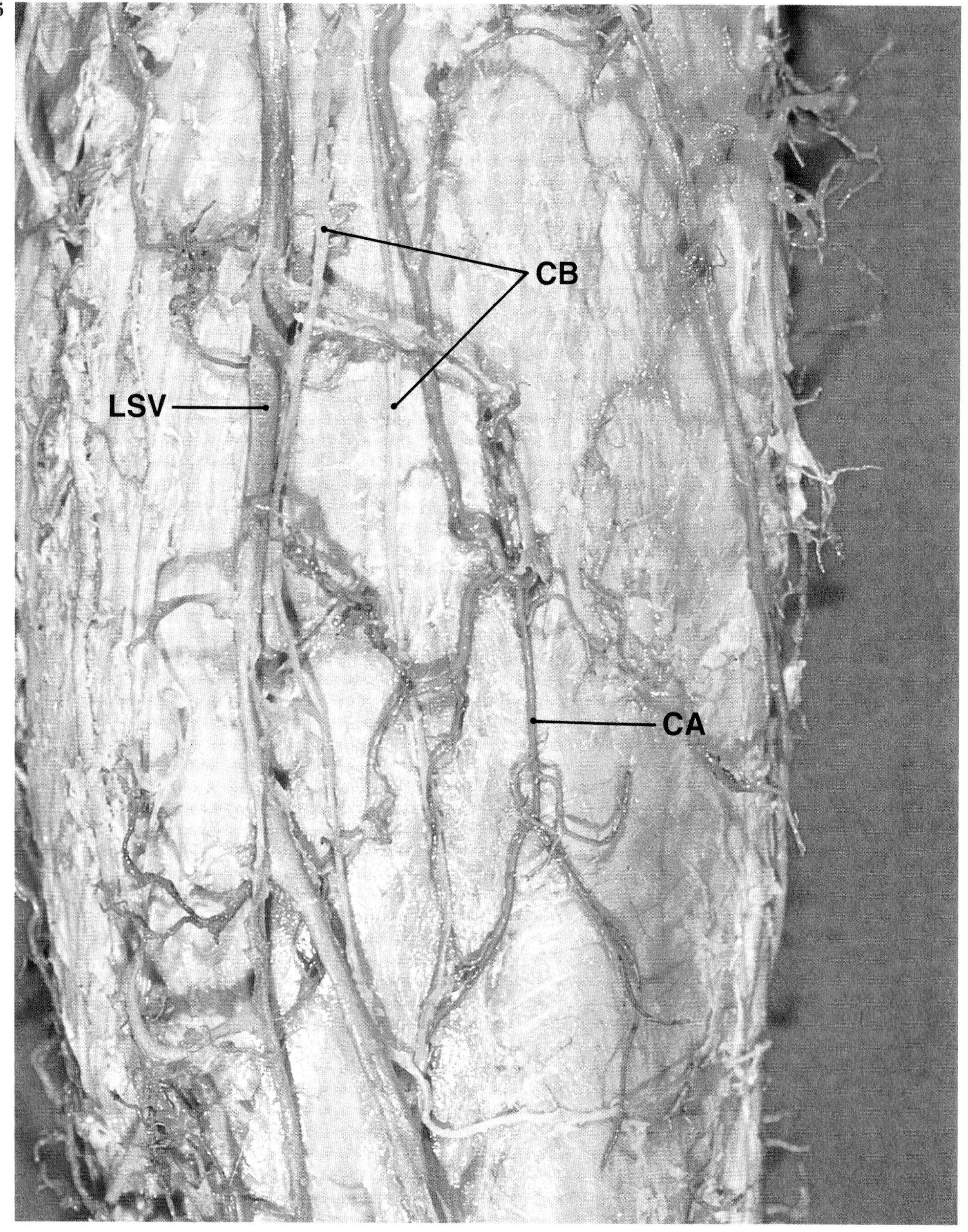

16: Epifascial arterial vessels (communicating arteries, CA) in a proximal lower medial leg. Long saphenous vein (LSV), cutaneous branches of the saphenous nerve (CB). Arterial tree injected with silicone rubber. (Orig. Prep. by DR. F. PLATZ, Anat. Instit., Freiburg)

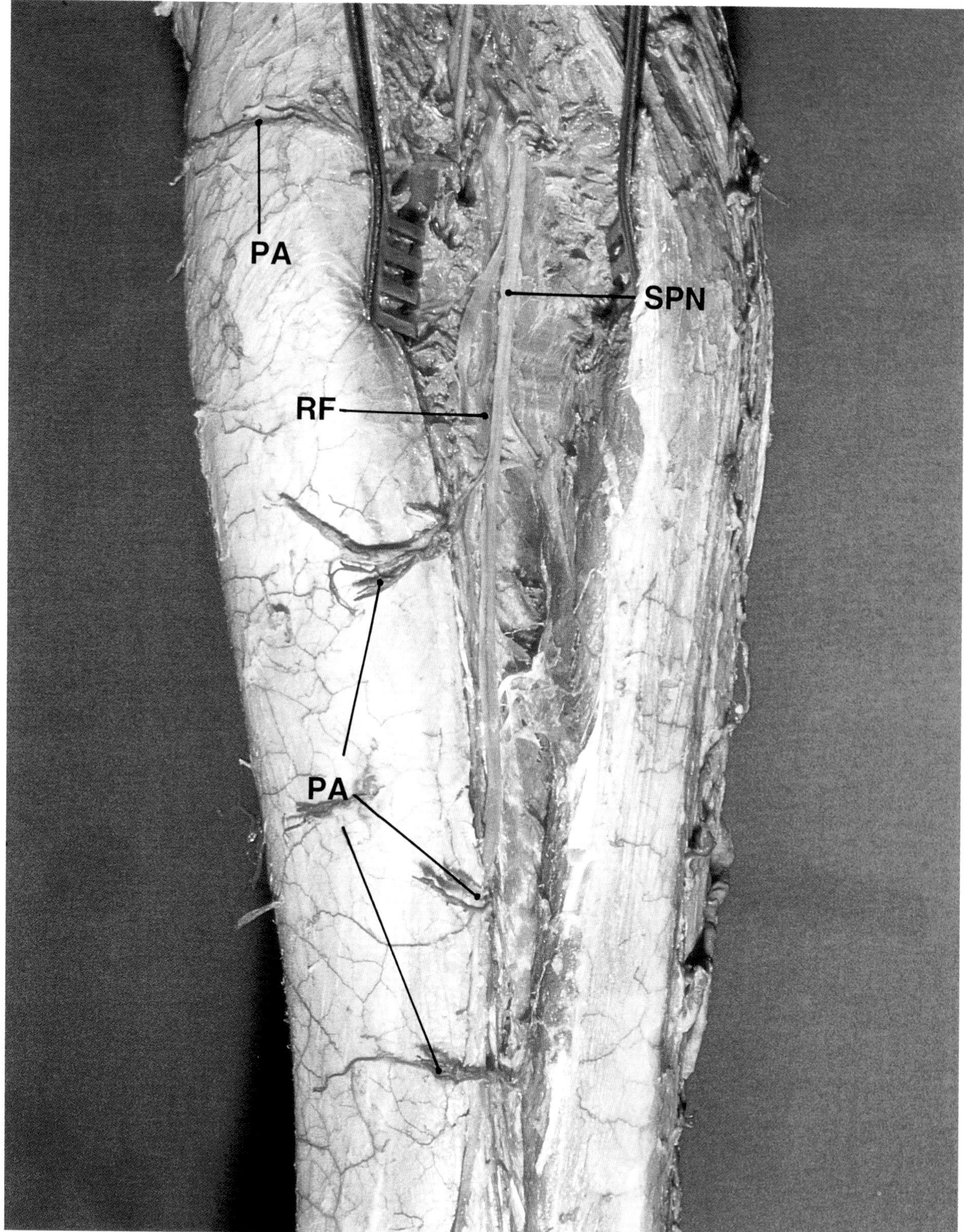

17: Dissected 'ramus fibularis' (RF, Hyrtl, 1864) of the anterior tibial artery, with a row of branching perforating arteries (PA) along the fibular side of the anterior intermuscular septum. SPN = superficial peroneal nerve. Arterial tree injected with red silicone rubber. (Orig. Prep. by DR. R. BAUMANN and DR. F. PLATZ, Anat. Instit., Freiburg)

18

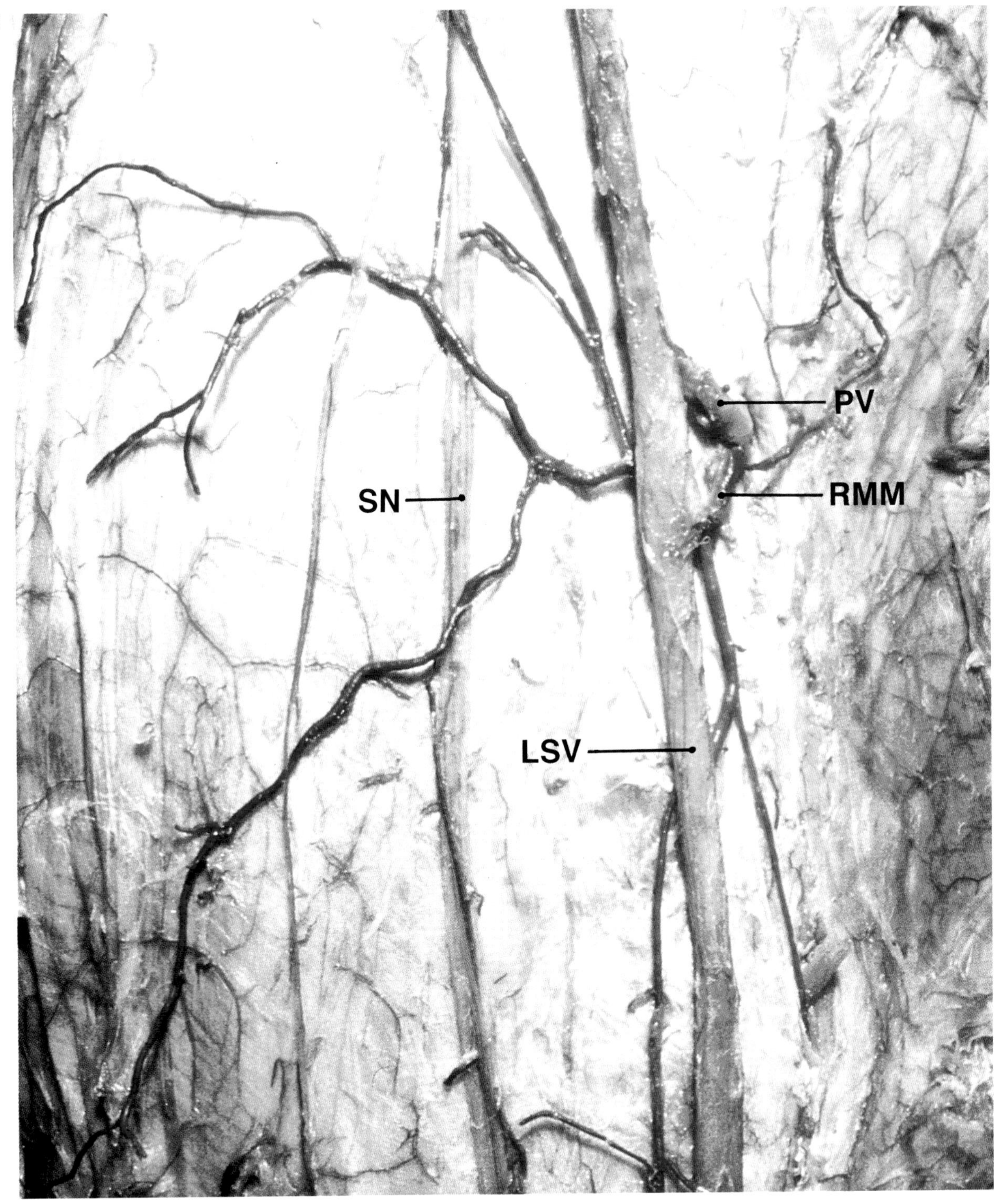

18: Lower medial leg with 'ramus musculocutaneous magnus' (RMM, 'great musculocutaneous branch', Baumann and Platz, 1987), 24.5 cm proximal to the medial malleolus. Take off from the posterior tibial artery 2.5 cm distal to the take off of the peroneal artery. Long saphenous vein (LSV) with anastomosing 'Sherman 24 cm' perforating vein (PV). SN = saphenous nerve. Arterial tree injected with red silicone rubber. (Orig. Prep. by Dr. R. Baumann and Dr. F. Platz, Anat. Instit., Freiburg)

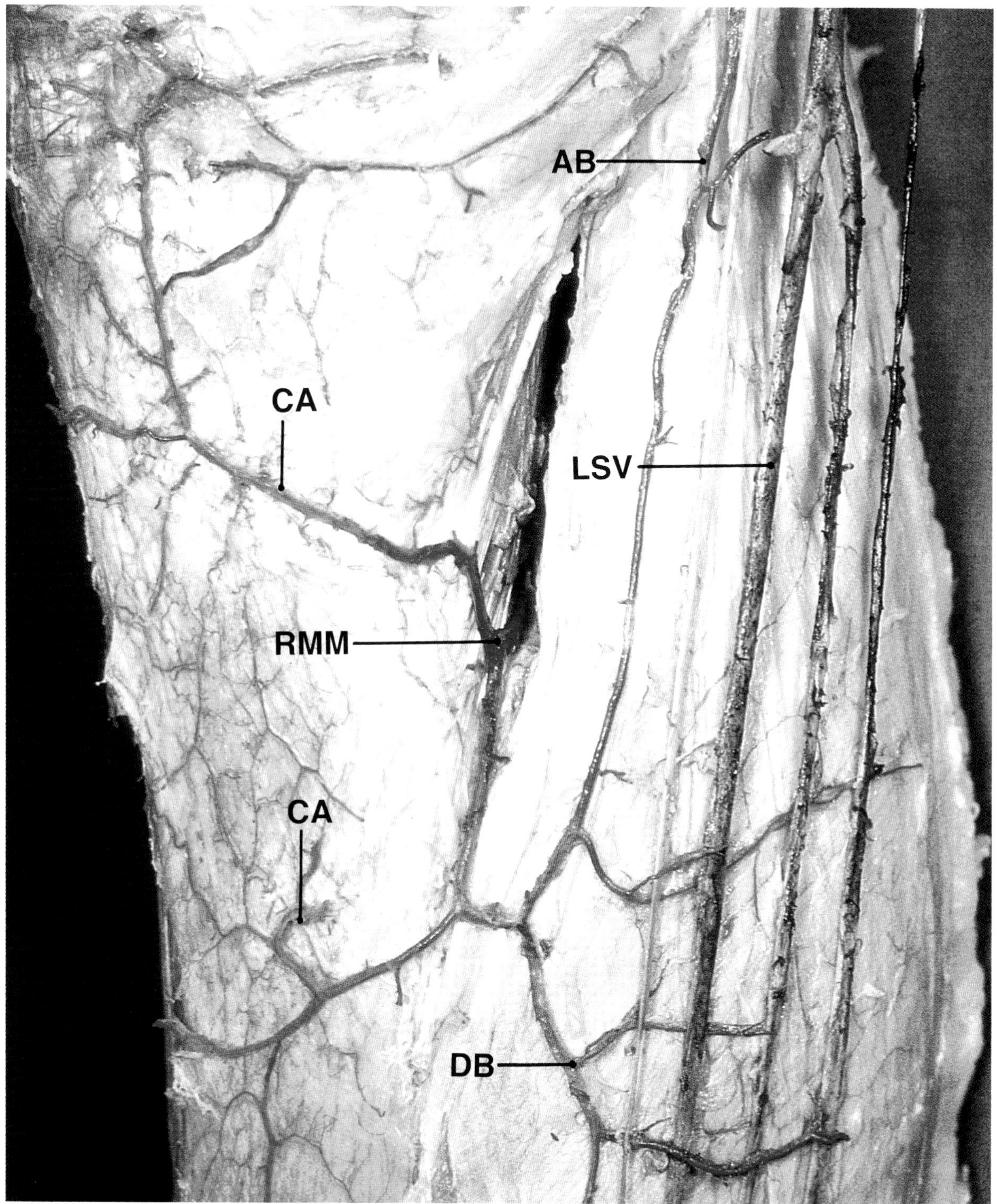

19: Well-developed 'ramus musculocutaneous magnus' (RMM), which has taken off from the 'truncus tibiofibularis' and penetrated the fascia with 2 branches, 4.5 cm and 8.5 cm distal to the tibial tuberosity. It branches in several directions via communicating arteries (CA). Ascending and descending branch (AB, DB) in the area of the long saphenous vein (LSV), which is in a somewhat posterior location. No topographical relationship to the Sherman or Boyd perforating vein is indicated. Arterial tree injected with red, proximally green, silicone rubber; large veins are blue. (Orig. Prep. by Dr. R. Baumann and Dr. F. Platz, Anat. Instit., Freiburg)

2. Phlebological conditions

Henner Altenkämper/Matthias Eldenburg

Types of varicose veins

Superficial venous system

20 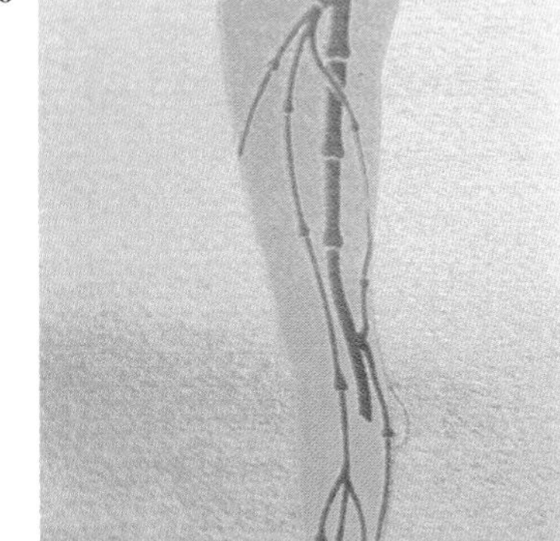

Truncal varicosis of long saphenous vein

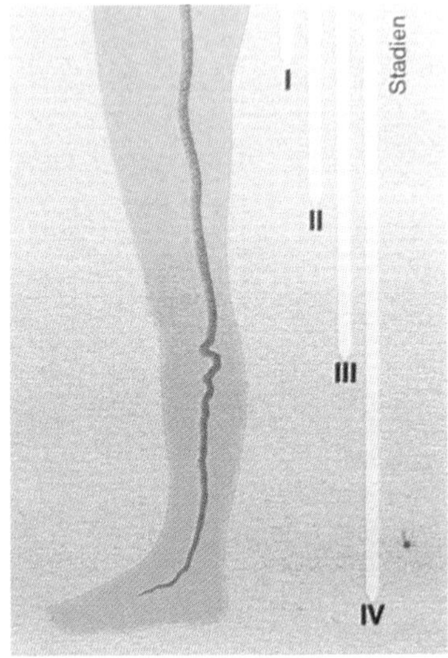

Truncal varicosis of short saphenous vein

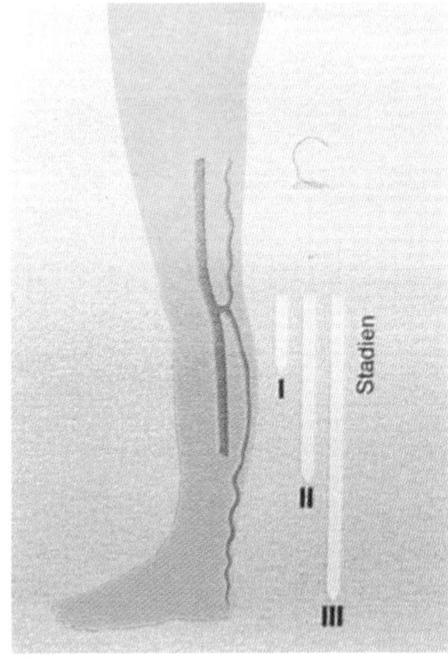

Tributary (branch) varicosis

21 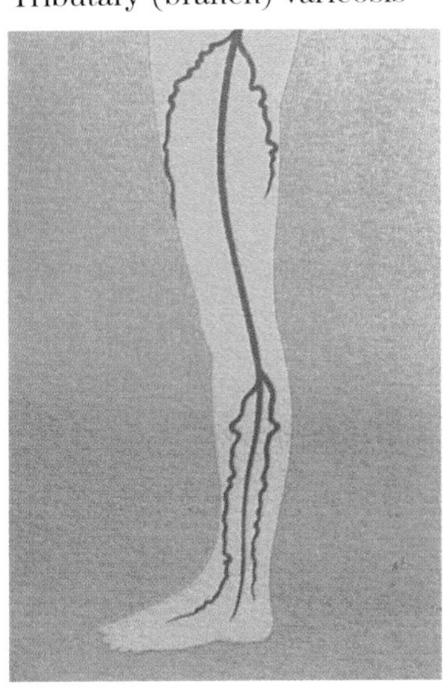

Reticular varicosis

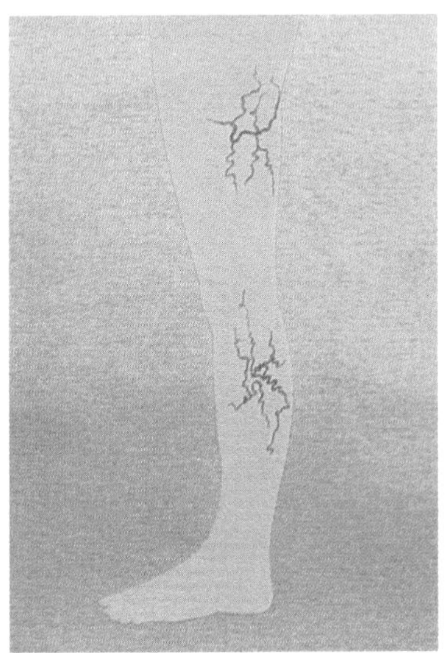

Perforator varicosis

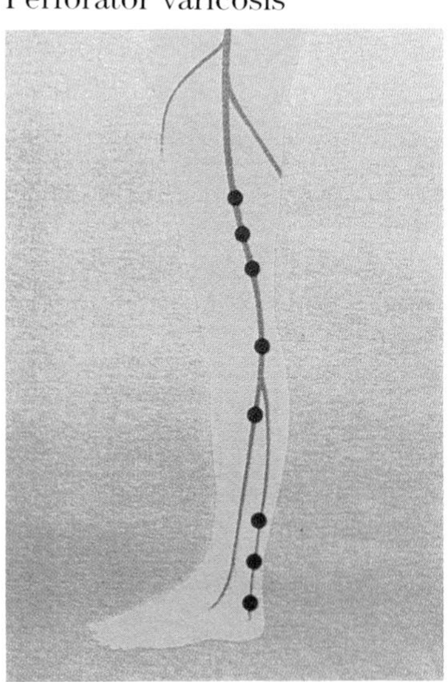

20/21: Varices are dilatations occurring over a shorter or longer distance in veins with irregular calibre, accompanied by typical changes of the vein wall and often with a disturbance of the centripetal propulsion function. These changes can occur in the superficial main trunks (truncal varicosis of the long saphenous or short saphenous vein), the branches, also called tributaries (branch varicosis), or small subcutaneous veins (reticular varicosis) as well as intradermal veins (spider vein varicosis). Incompetent perforator veins can also lead to a varicosis of subcutaneous or intradermal veins (perforator varicosis).

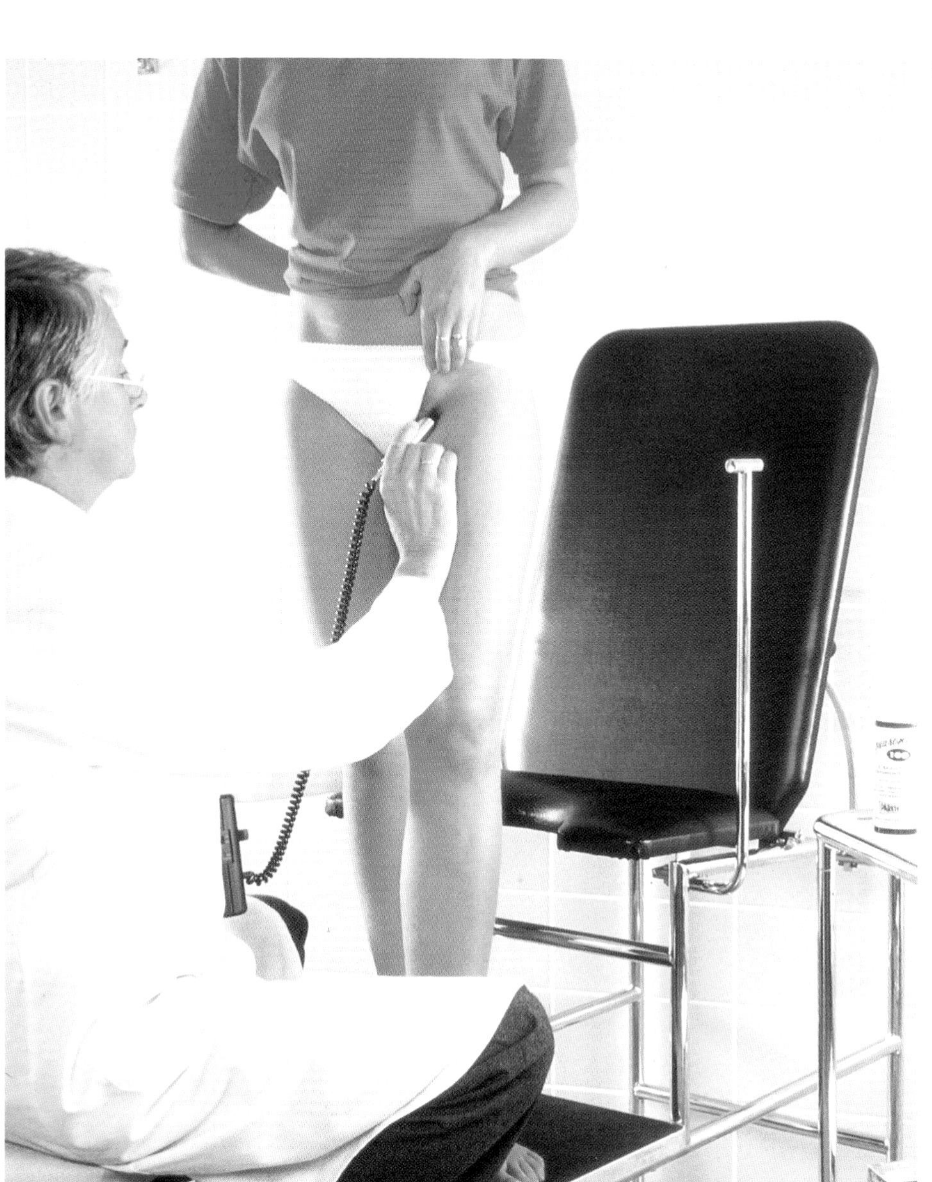

22: On the basis of Doppler findings, a trunk varicosis can be divided into a complete and an incomplete form. In complete trunk varicosis, there is a reflux over the saphenofemoral junction (junction of the long saphenous vein and femoral vein), which with the Doppler probe can be traced distally along the trunk. In incomplete trunk varicosis, the reflux of venous blood, during a Valsalva manoeuvre, is demonstrable only at a certain distance from the saphenofemoral junction (e.g. trunk varicosis on basis of incompetence of a Dodd perforator in the thigh). The Hach classification divides a complete trunk varicosis of the long saphenous vein in four stages depending on the location of the distal point of incompetence; this classification can be used as a basis for therapeutic decision making. In Stage I, the reflux can be demonstrated down to a few centimeters below the saphenofemoral junction; in Stage II it extends down to the distal thigh, in Stage III to the middle of the lower leg, and in Stage IV the most distal point of incompetence is at the ankle level.

23

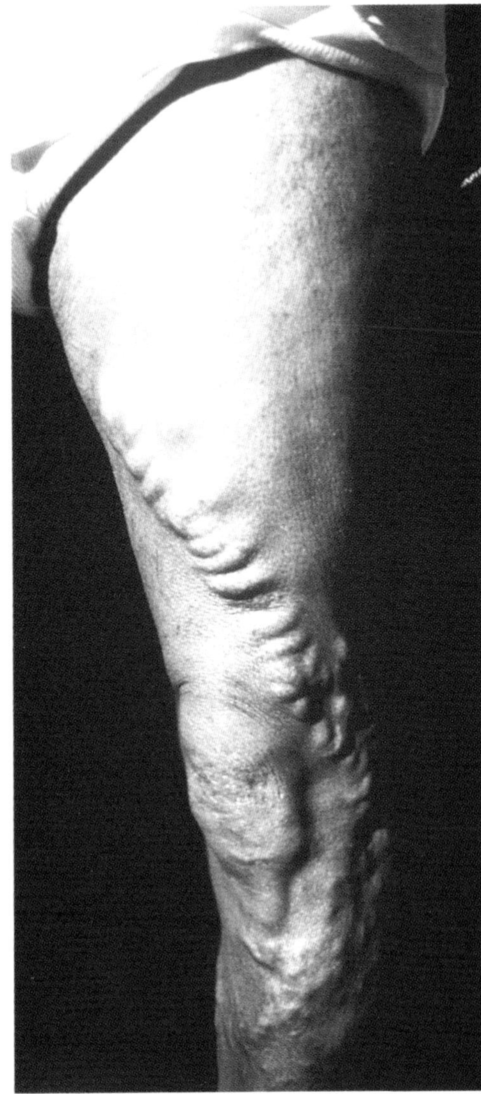

24

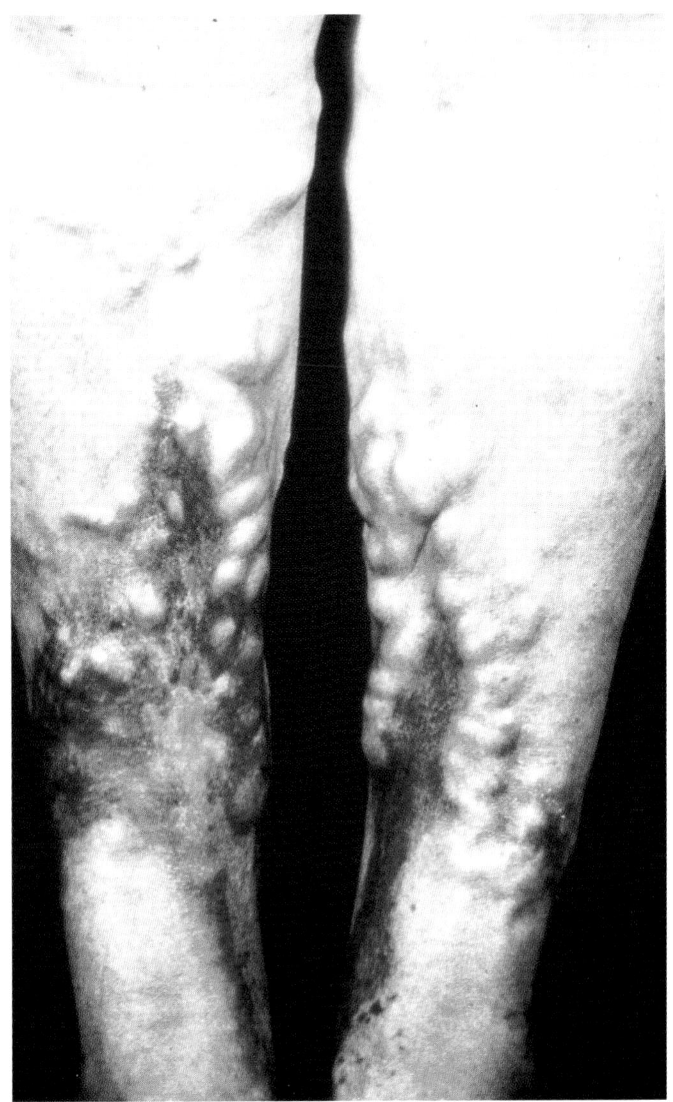

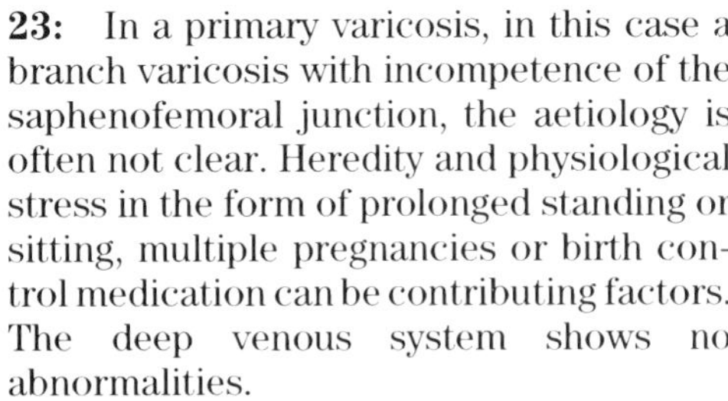

23: In a primary varicosis, in this case a branch varicosis with incompetence of the saphenofemoral junction, the aetiology is often not clear. Heredity and physiological stress in the form of prolonged standing or sitting, multiple pregnancies or birth control medication can be contributing factors. The deep venous system shows no abnormalities.

24: A secondary varicosis is most often the result of thrombosis of the deep veins. But other causes of occlusion or stenosis of the deep venous system have to be mentioned, such as an abdominal or pelvic tumour, arteriovenous fistulas, and other causes. A special form is the so-called dependency syndrome, in which the varicosis is caused by incompetence of the venous muscle pump, e.g. on the basis of arthritic changes of the ankle joint. The picture shows a severe post-thrombotic syndrome with secondary varicosis.

25

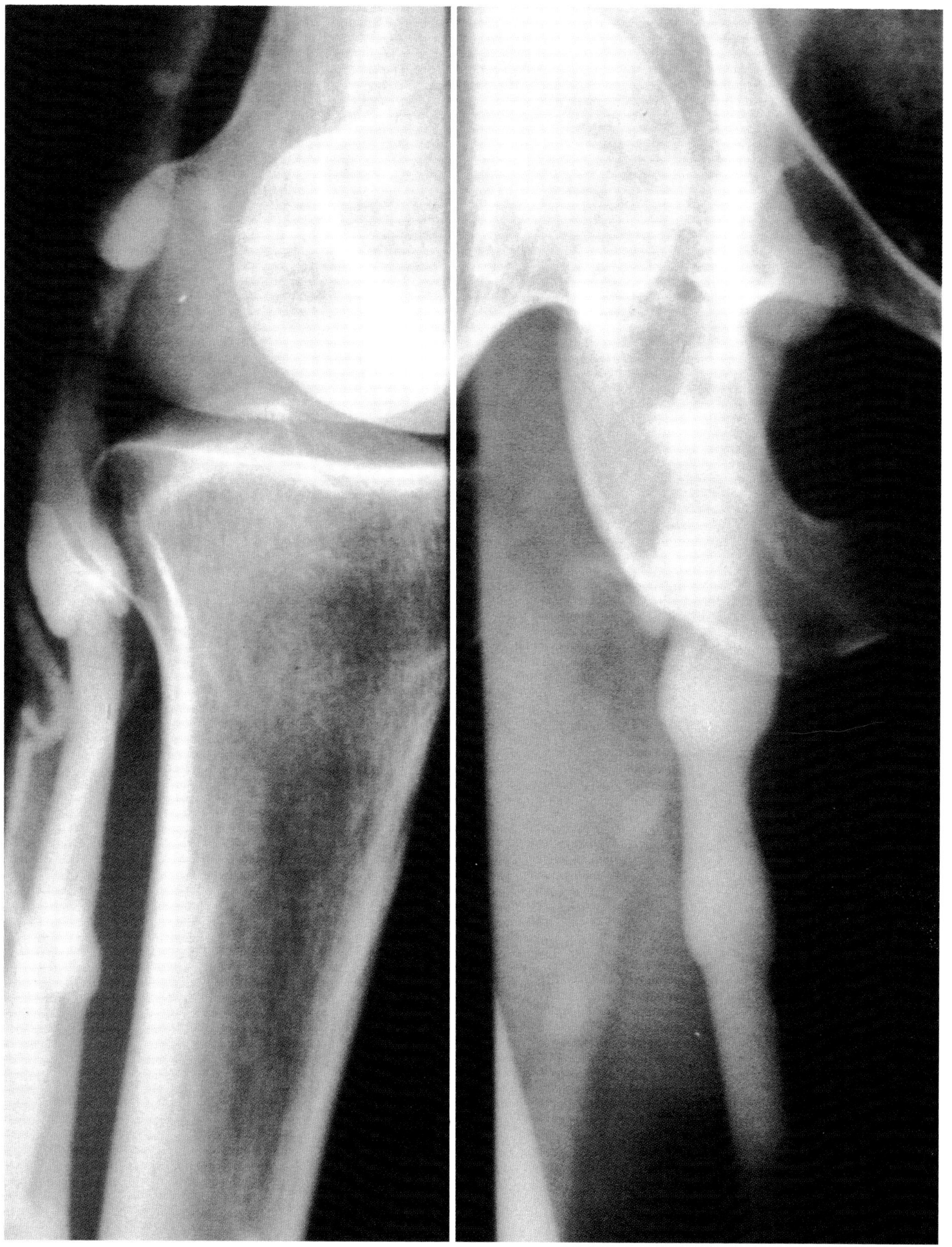

25: Venogram of an intact venous system with clearly recognizable valves in the deep veins. The long saphenous vein is not visualized because of competence of the valve at the saphenofemoral junction.

26

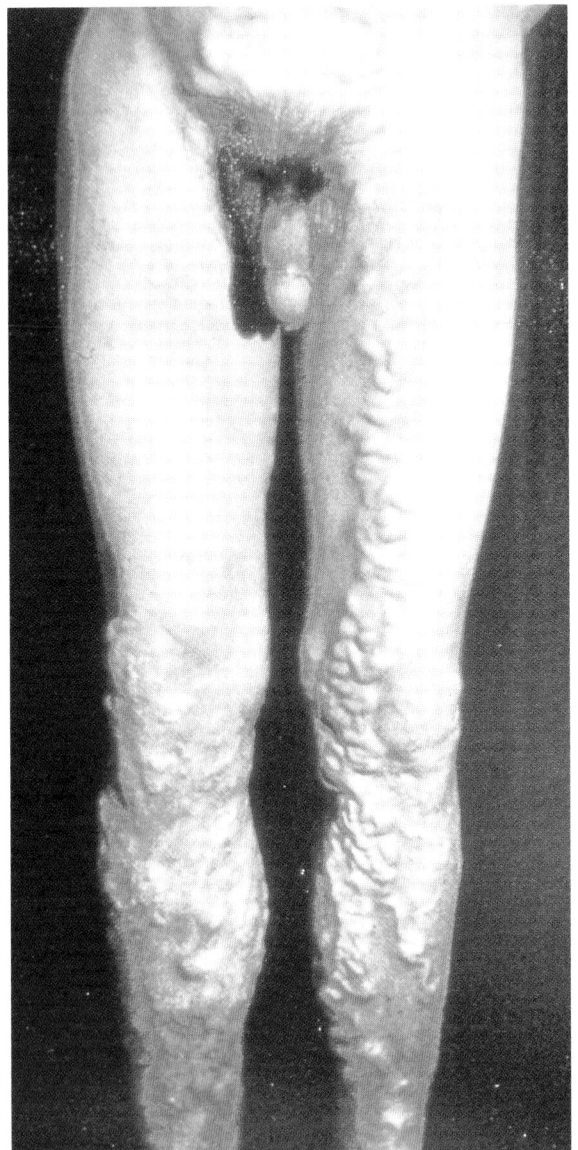

27

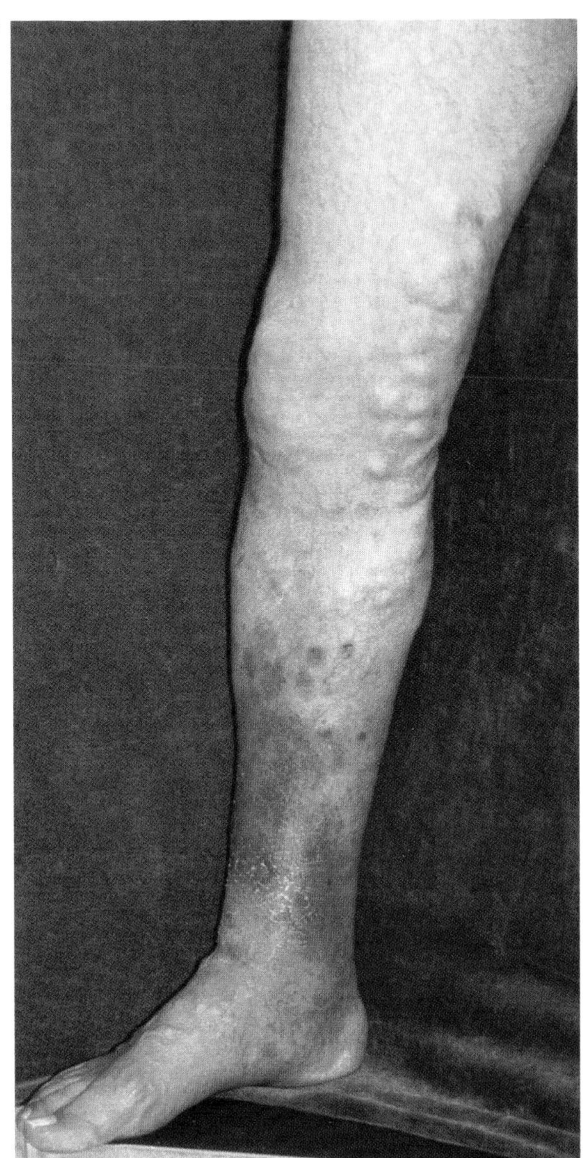

26: Massive varicosis of the lower extremity and abdominal wall. Although the leg varicosis could represent a primary form, the varices of the superficial epigastric veins indicate a venous obstruction in the pelvis, and therefore have to be interpreted as secondary varices.

27: Trunk varicosis of the long saphenous vein with clearly evident trophic changes in the lower leg (chronic venous insufficiency Stage III with ulcerations in the area of the distal anterior tibia).

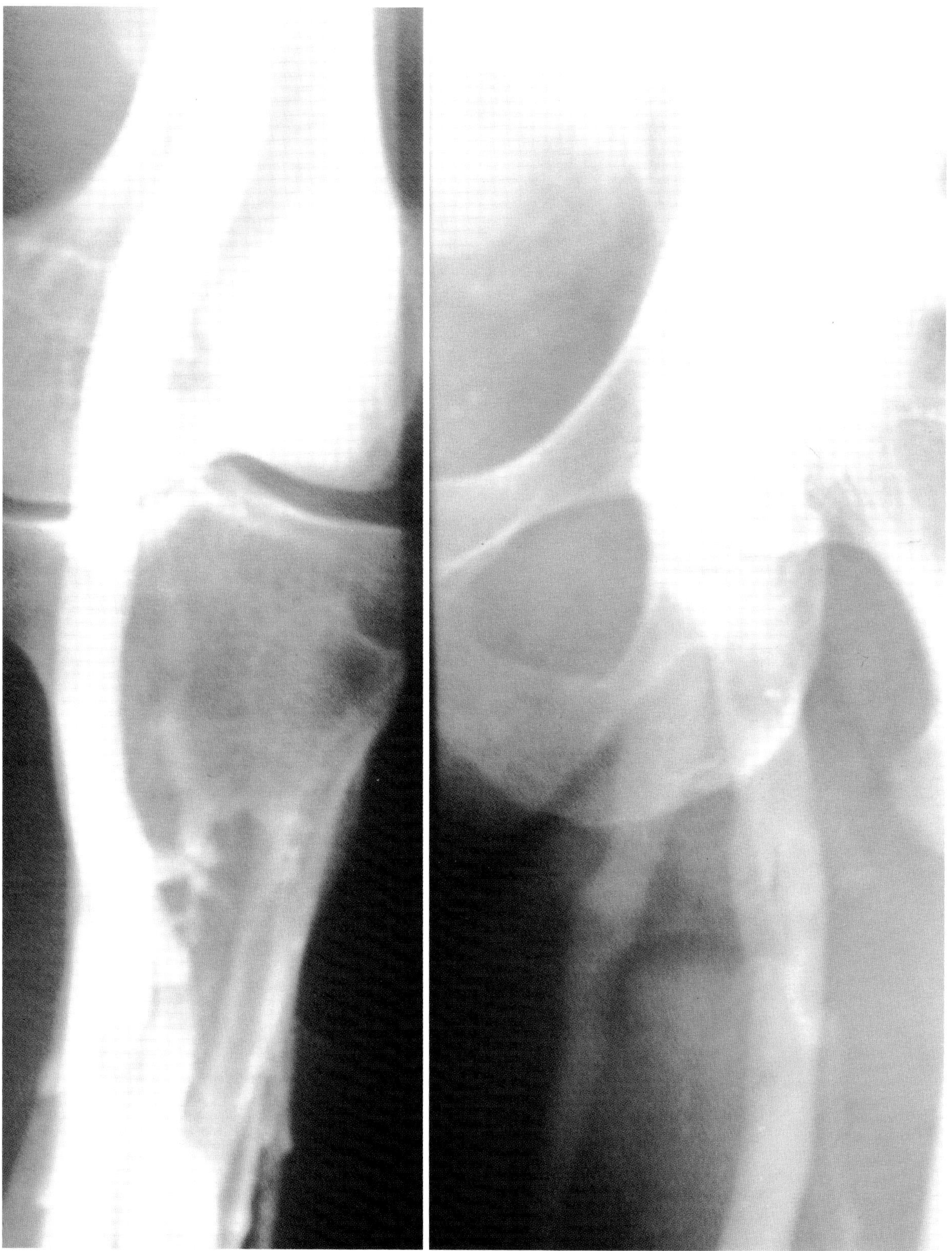

28: In this ascending venogram, the long saphenous vein is visualized because of incompetence of the saphenofemoral junction. The so-called telescope phenomenon of the normal long saphenous vein (changes in calibre at the valves from proximal to distal) is missing.

29

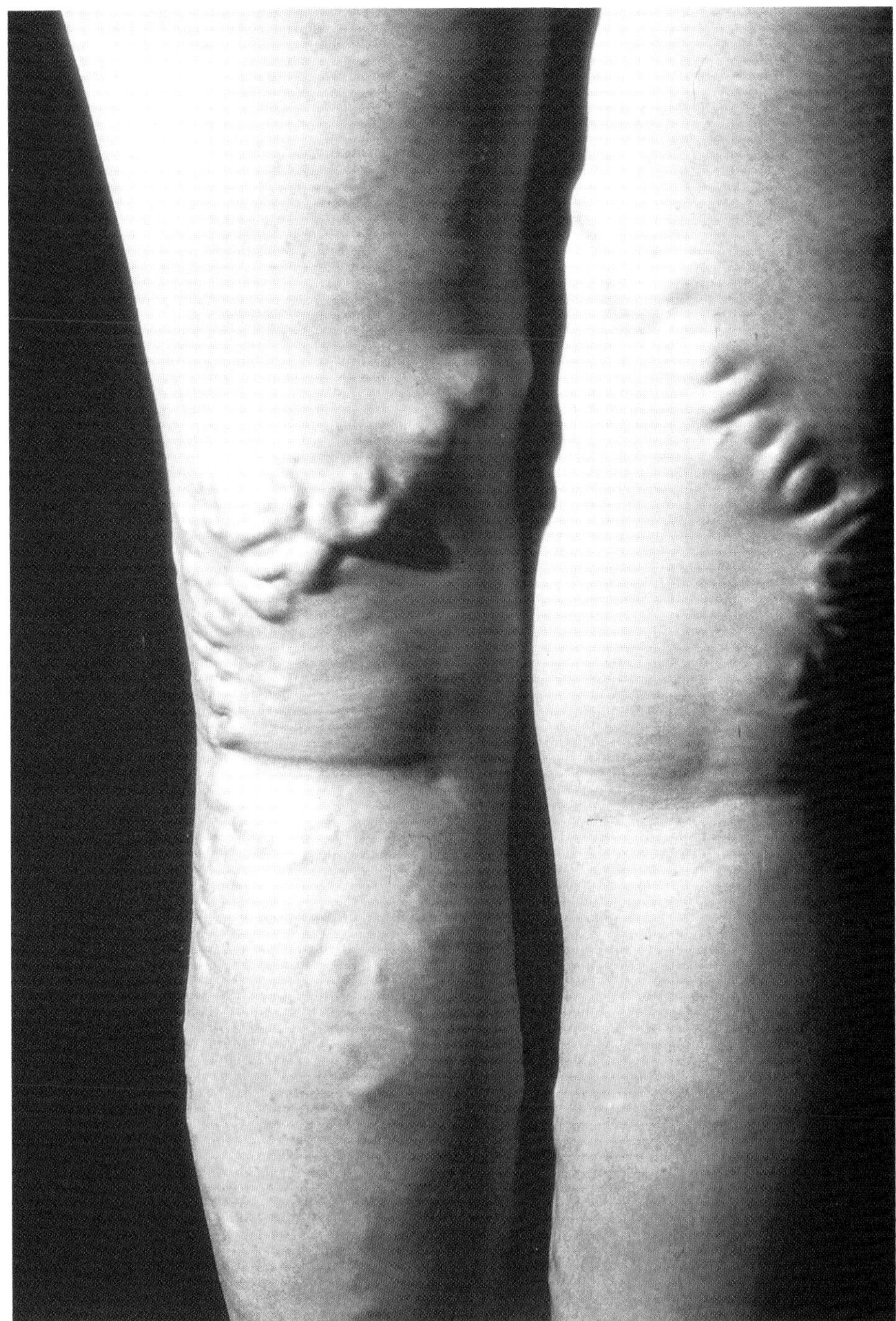

29: Varicosis of the posterior saphenous vein, which courses towards the lateral side of the popliteal fossa.

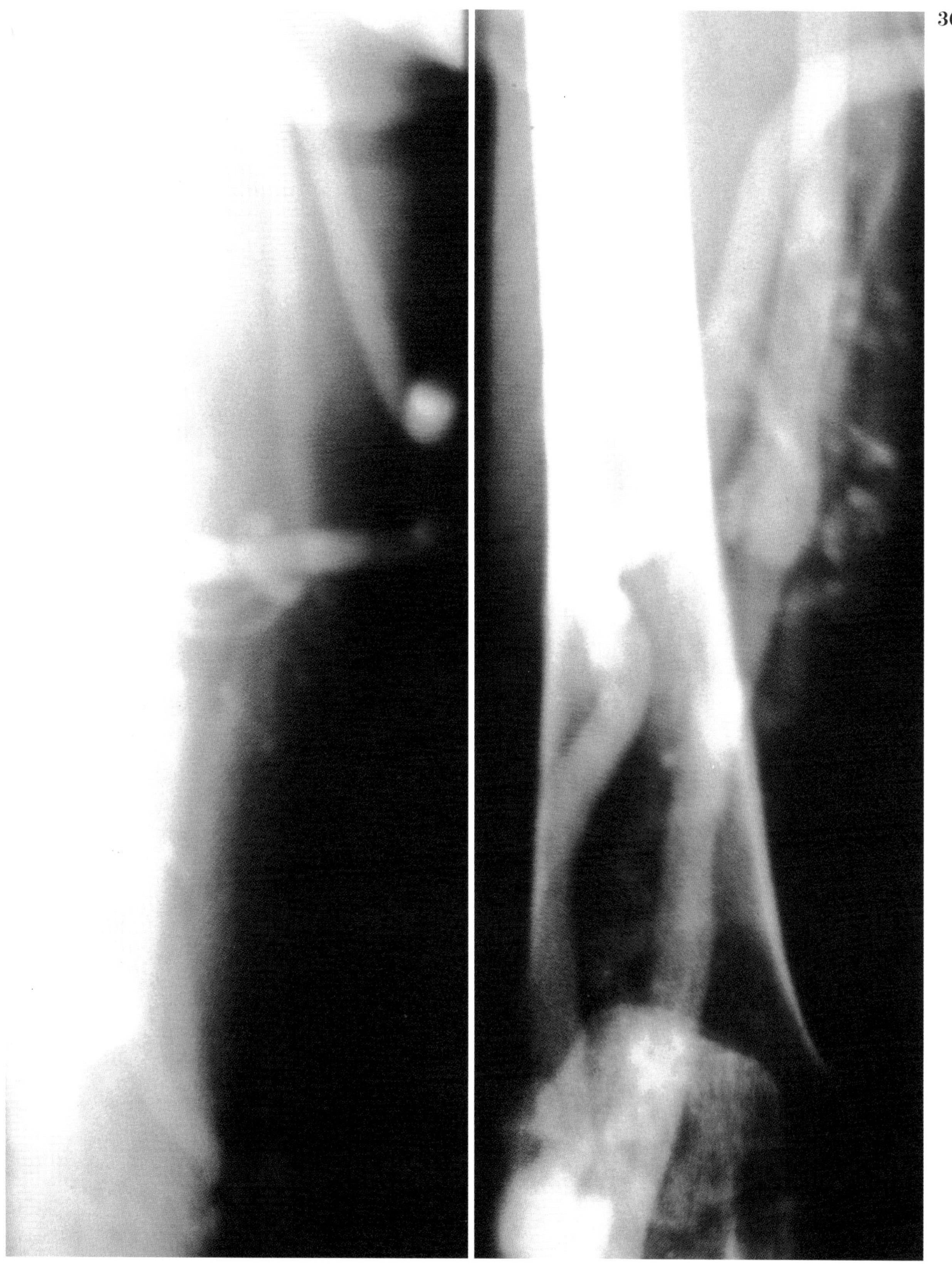

30

30: Venogram of the anastomotic vein of Giacomini.

31

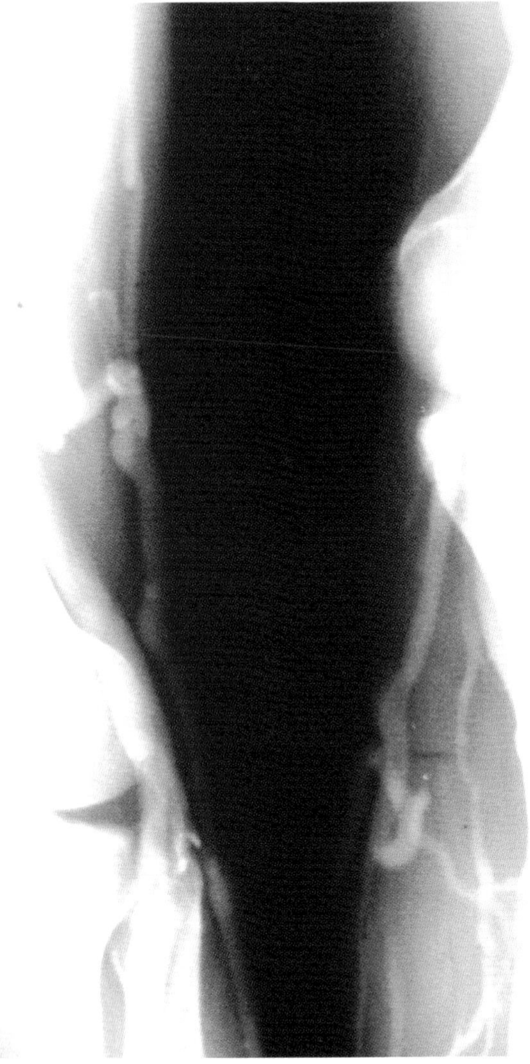

32

31: There is great anatomical variability in the junction of the short saphenous vein and the deep venous system. This venogram shows the short saphenous vein joining at a considerable distance above the popliteal fossa.

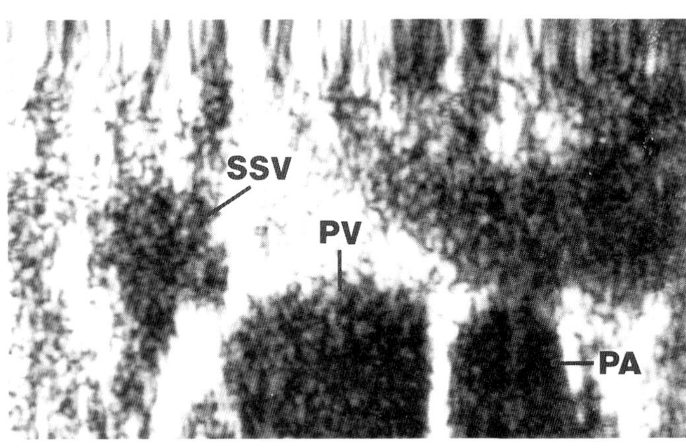

32: Incompetent short saphenous vein (*above*) with clearly visible ectasia near the junction with the deep venous system. Duplex ultrasonography (*below*) can also be used to visualize the saphenopopliteal junction. SSV: short saphenous vein. PV: popliteal vein. PA: popliteal artery.

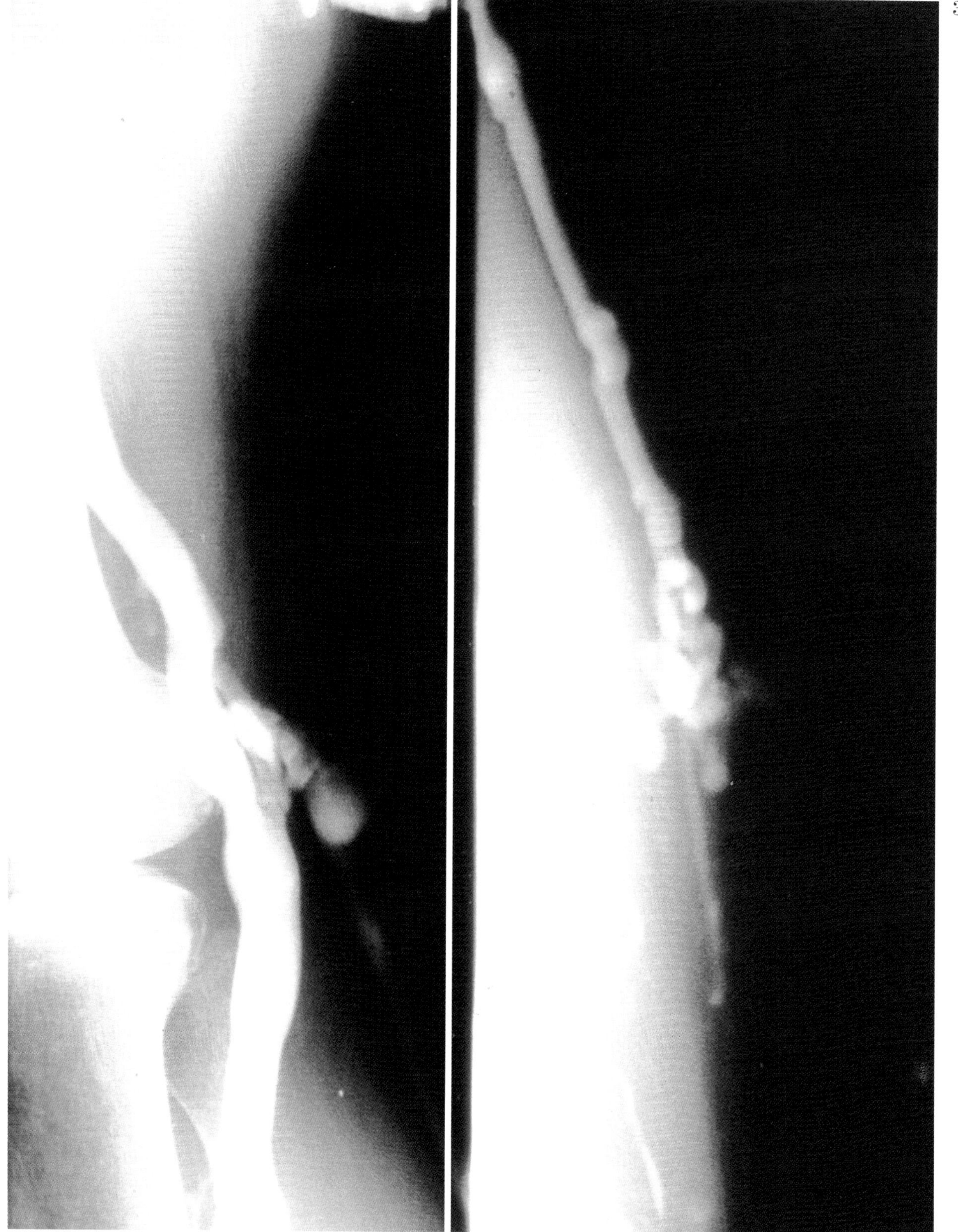

33

33: Varicosis of the short saphenous vein. Depending on the severity, the treatment consists of surgical ligation and division with stripping or sclerotherapy.

34

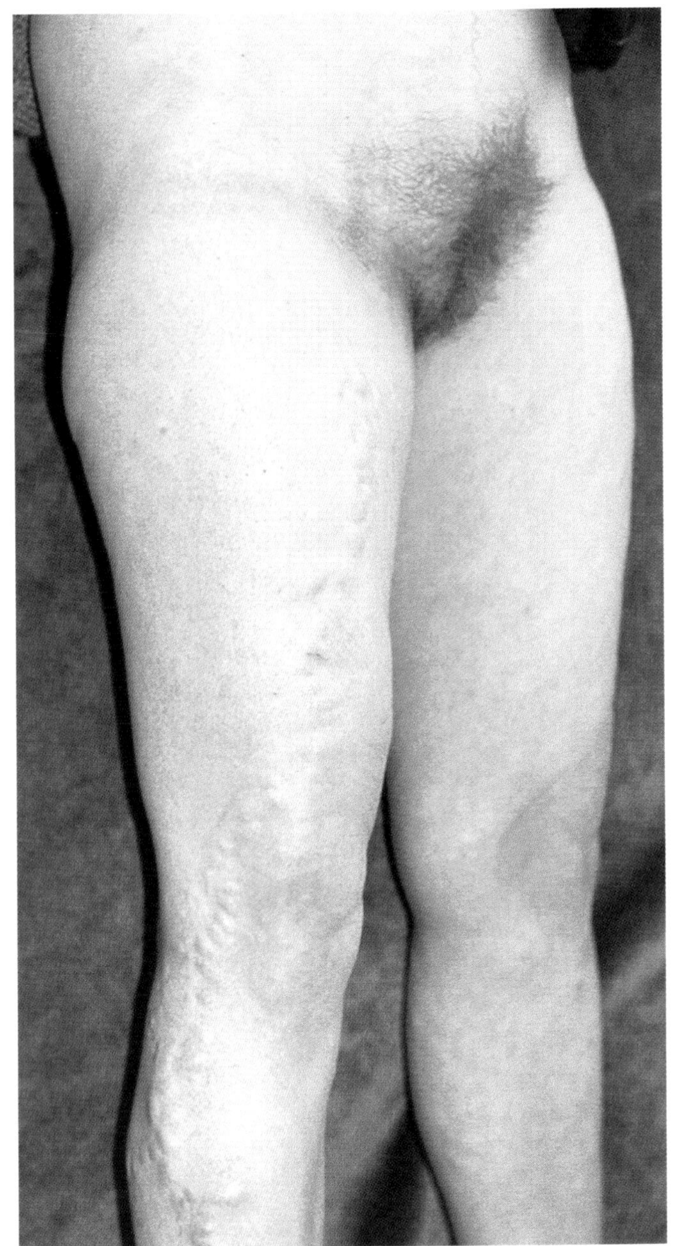

34: Marked branch varicosis of the anterior saphenous vein caused by incompetence of the saphenofemoral junction.

35

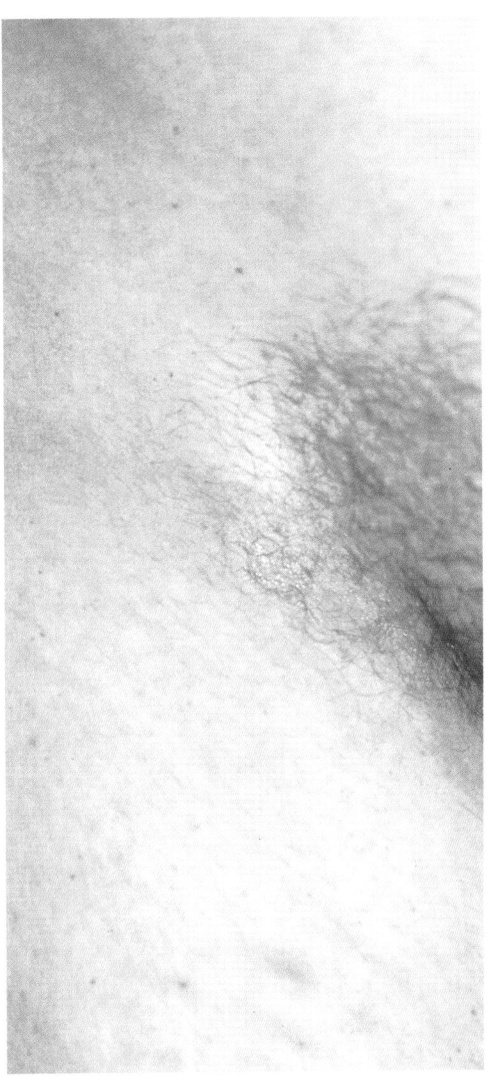

35: A close-up of the inguinal region of this patient shows a venous aneurysm of the long saphenous vein due to venous hypertension at the saphenofemoral junction.

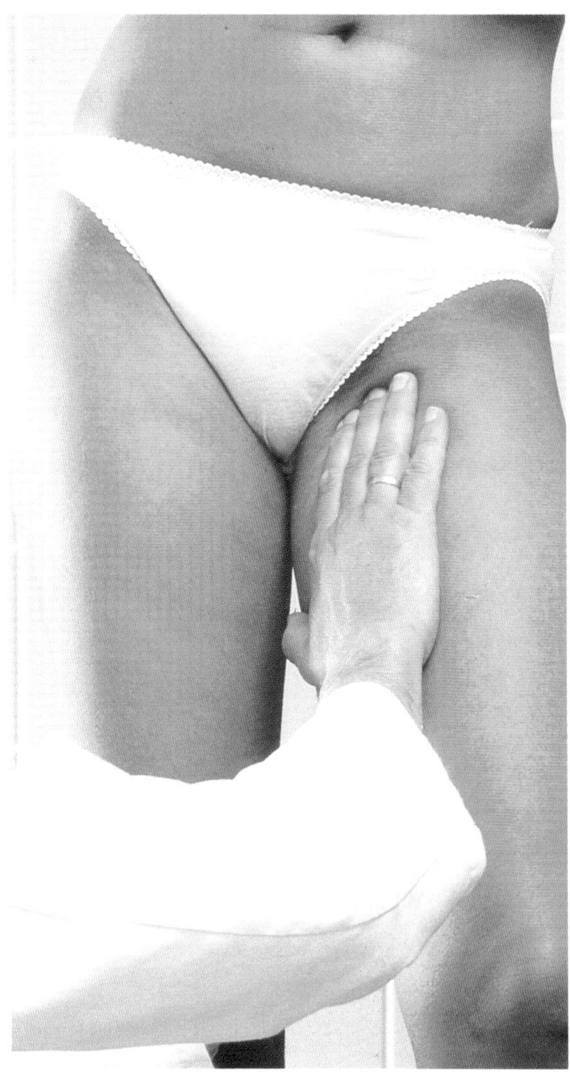

36: A palpable thrill in the groin area when the patient performs a Valsalva manoeuvre or coughs indicates valve incompetence at the sapheno-femoral junction.

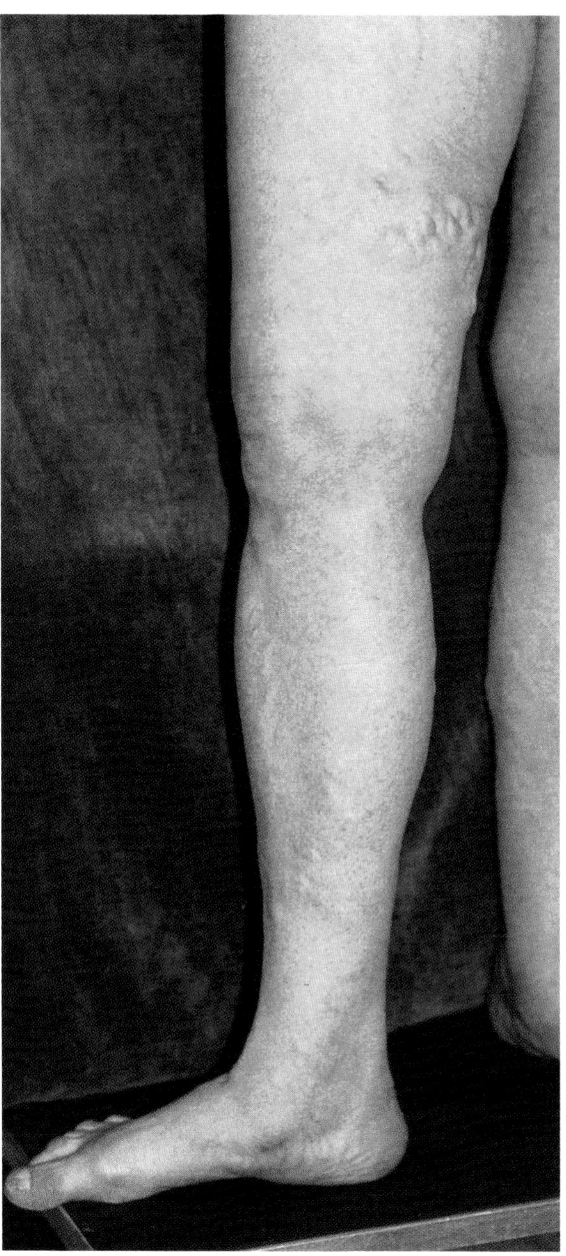

37: The main finding in this patient is incomplete truncal varicosis from an incompetent Dodd perforator of the right leg combined with a less pronounced varicosis in the area of the anterior crural vein, which probably is also caused by incompetent perforators.

38

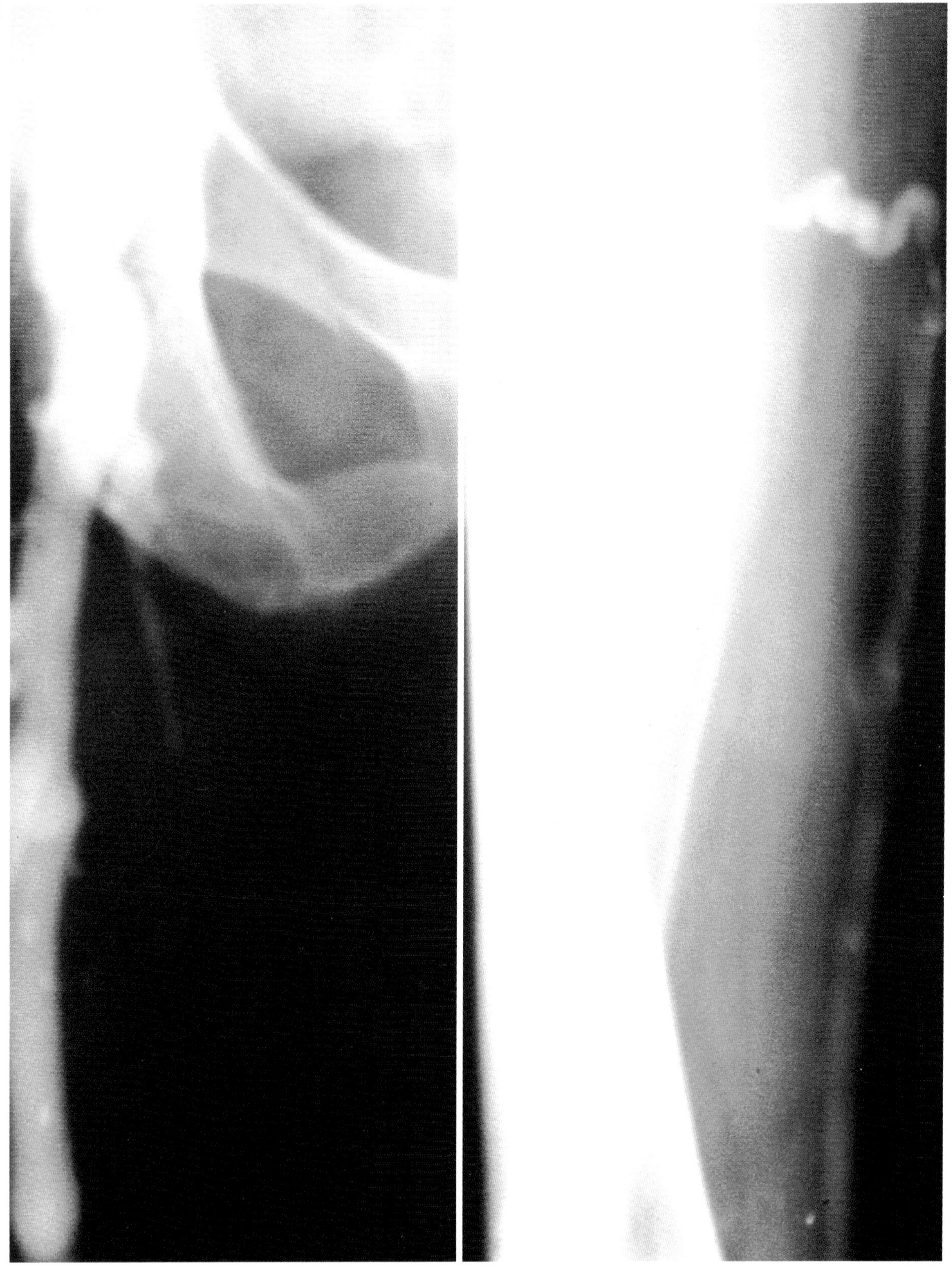

38: In this patient, in addition to an early incompetence of the long saphenous vein, an incomplete truncal varicosis is seen caused by an incompetent Dodd perforator.

39

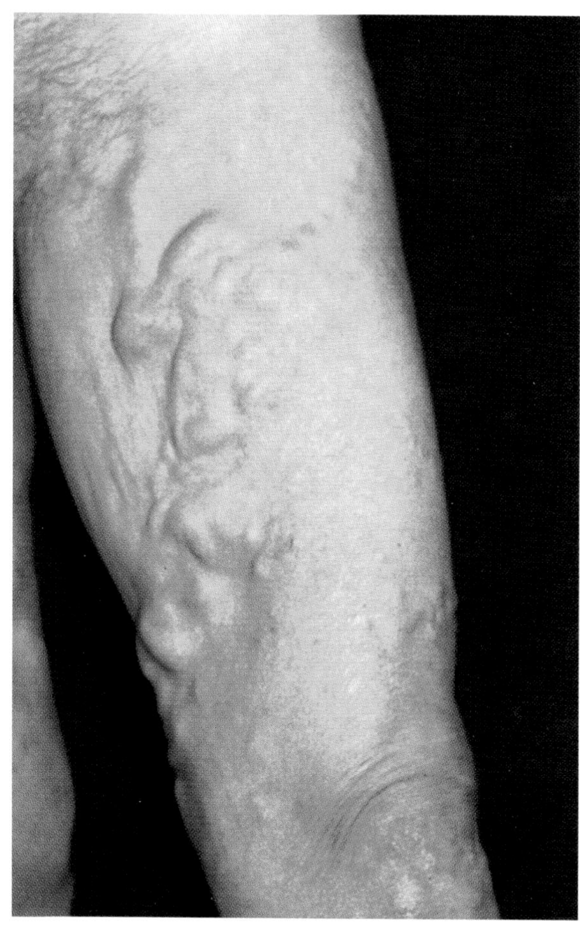

39: A complete truncal varicosis which led to markedly convoluted varicosities of the upper leg.

41

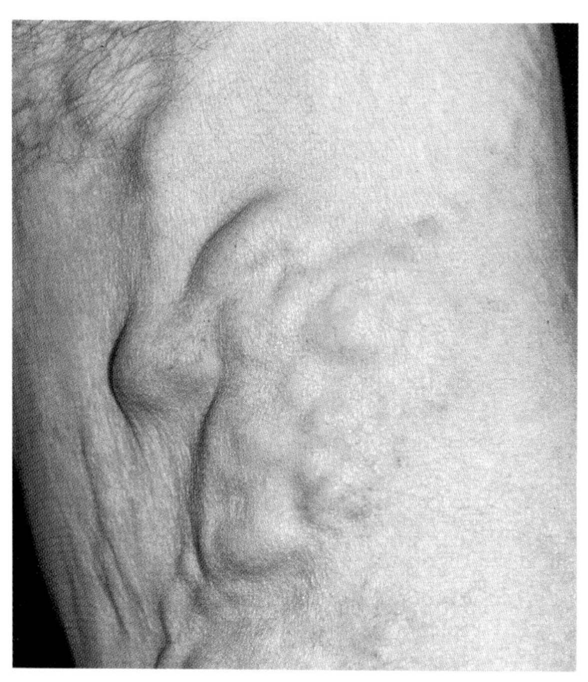

40

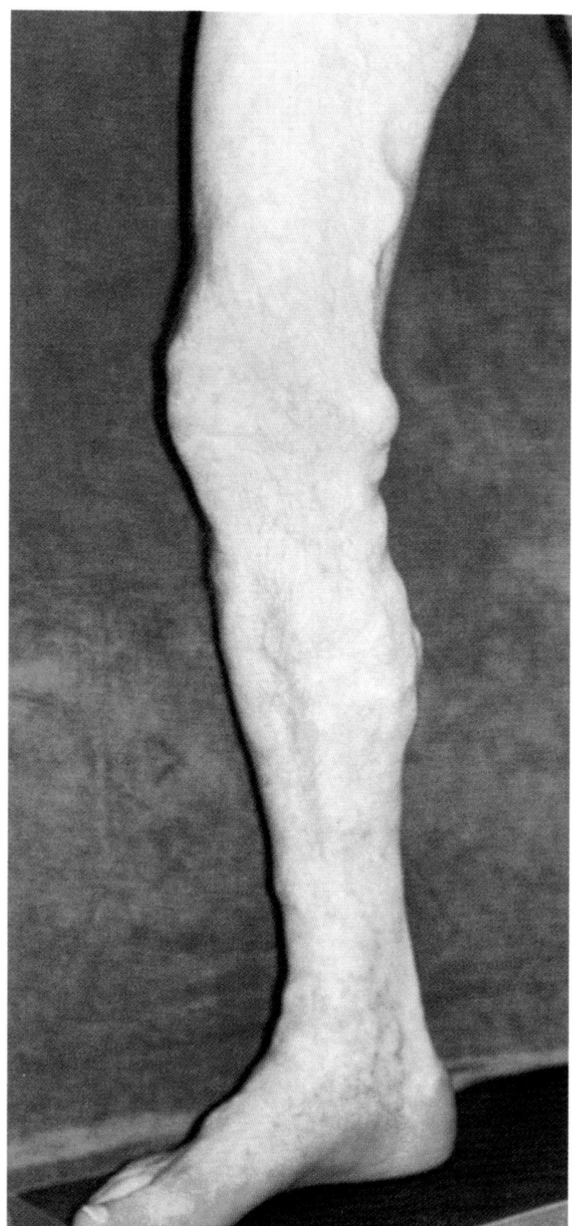

40: A combination of truncal varicosis and secondarily incompetent perforator veins is not an infrequent finding. Fine veins near the medial margin of the foot form a corona phlebectatica paraplantaris, which is a sign of chronic stage 1 venous insufficiency.

41: Because of the venous dilatations and the many vessels entering this varicose area, the marked incompetence of the saphenofemoral junction cannot be treated with sclerotherapy. Only a ligation and division combined with stripping of the long saphenous vein can take care of the venous insufficiency.

42

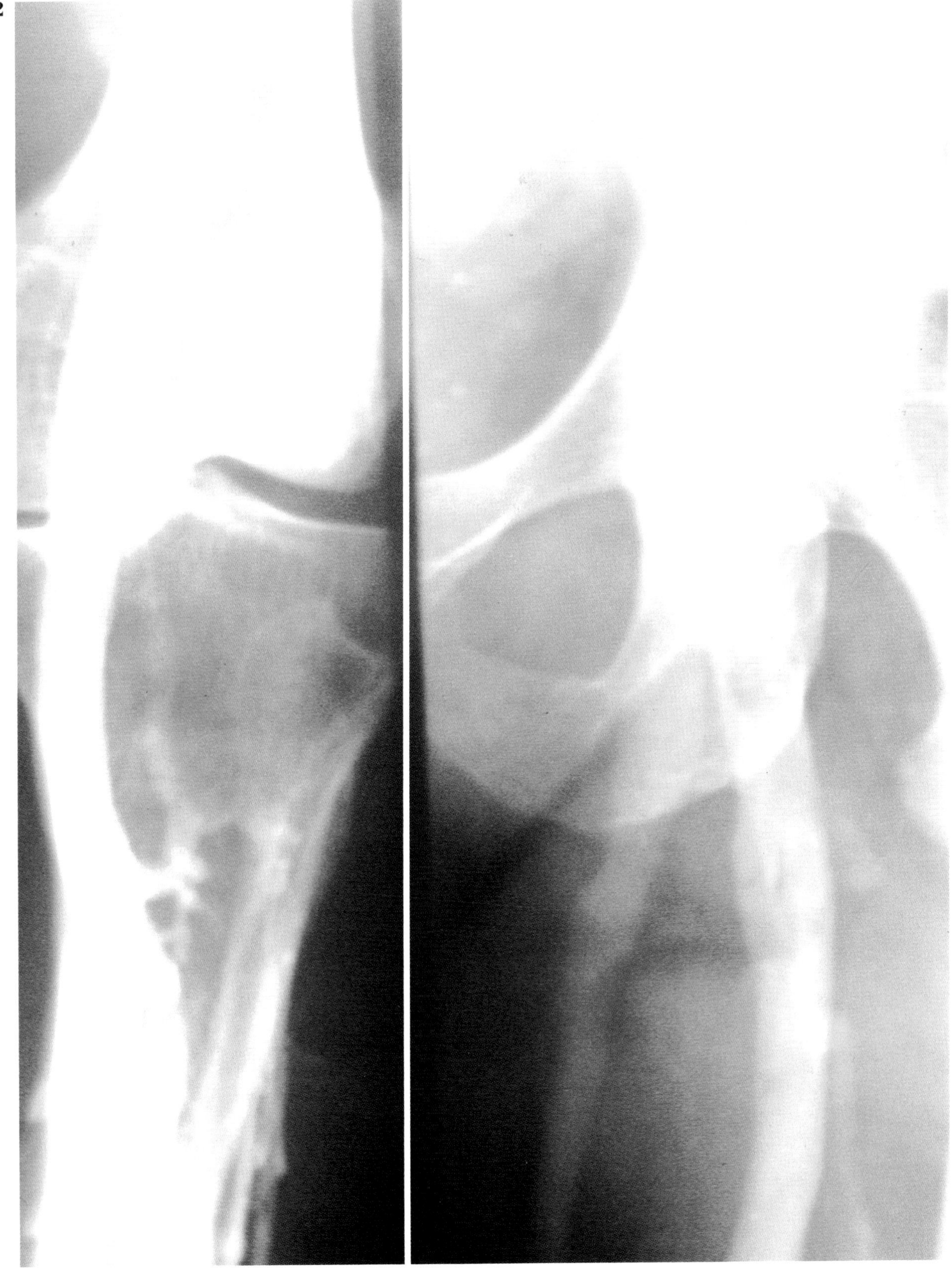

42: Kinking of the popliteal vein in a secondary femoropopliteal incompetence.

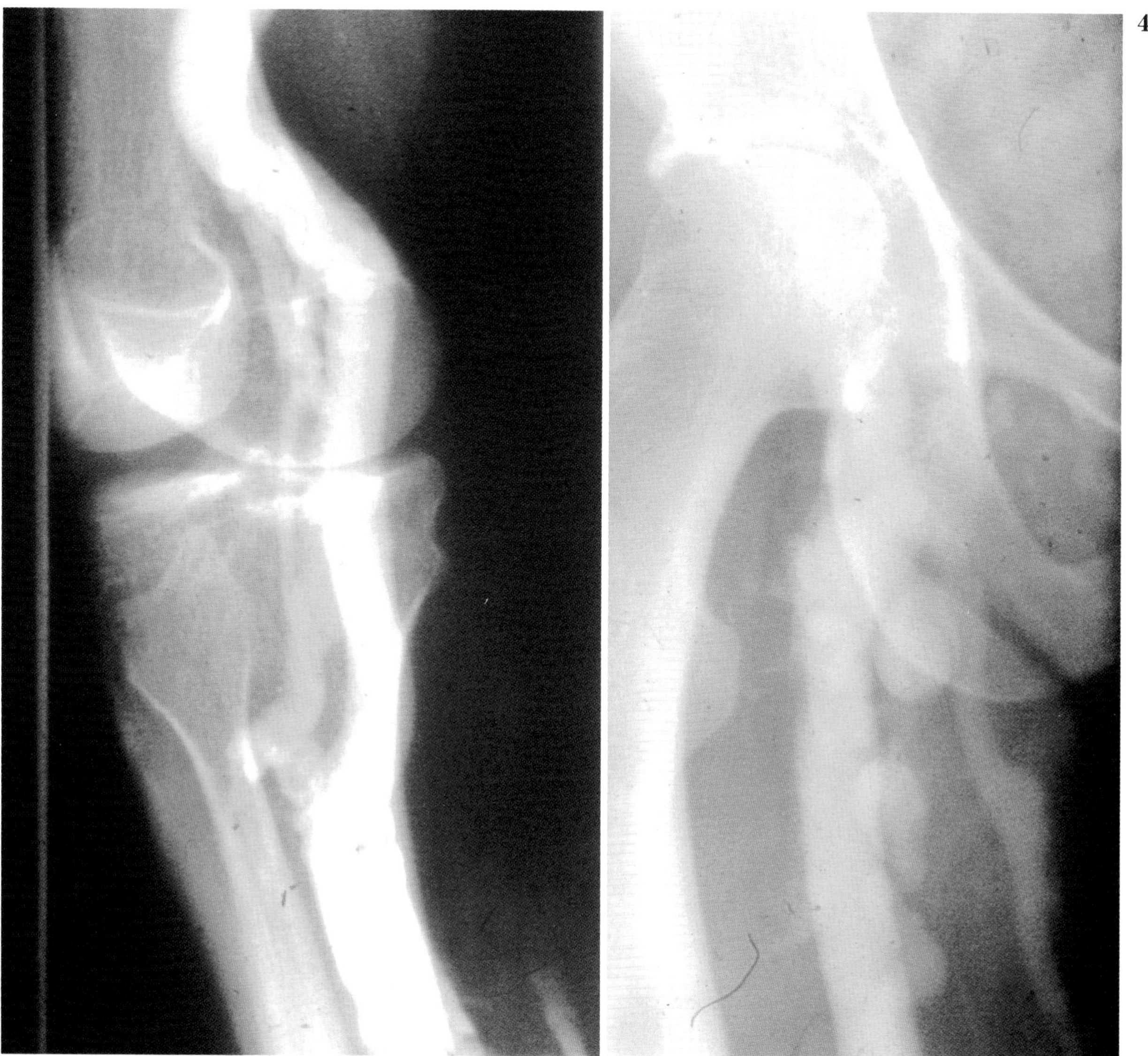

43: A truncal varicosis can lead to secondary femoropopliteal incompetence. This ascending pressure venogram shows an incompetent long saphenous vein and clearly dilated superficial femoral and popliteal vein with valve incompetence and elongation of the latter.

44

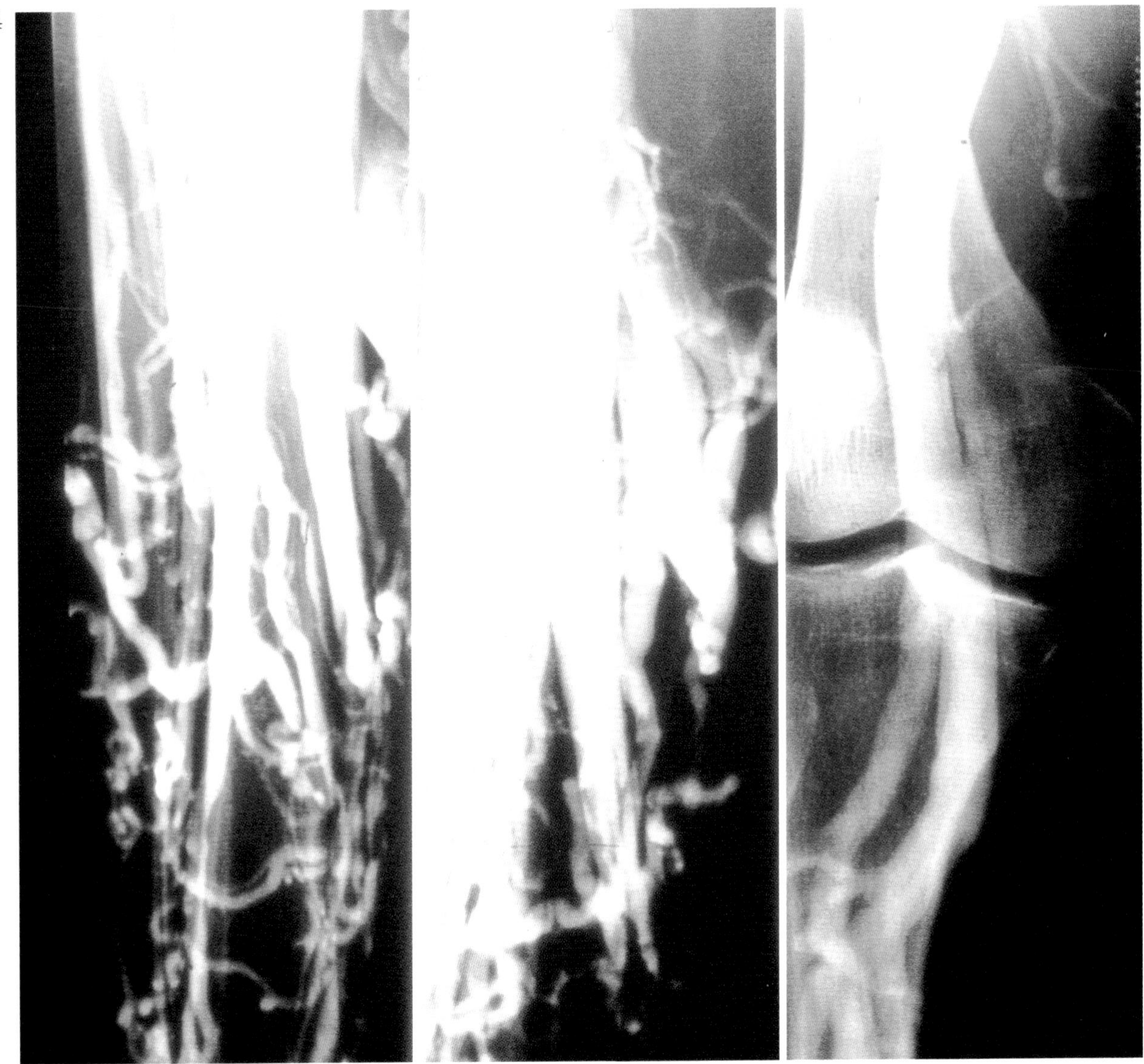

44: This is a case of short saphenous vein incompetence with only moderate dilatation of the popliteal vein but marked dilatation of the deep veins of the lower leg and calf veins, indicating the distal type of a secondary deep vein incompetence.

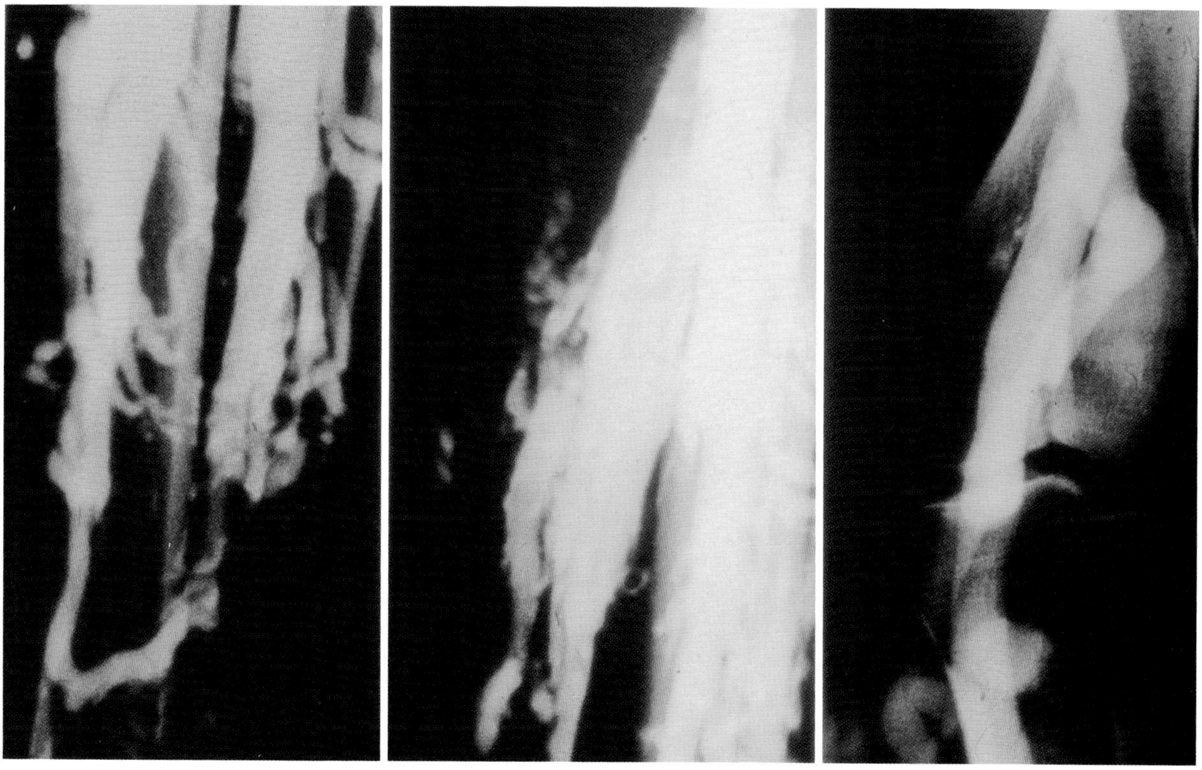

45: Marked incompetence of the deep and calf veins of the lower leg.

46: The retrograde flow from the deep to the superficial venous system causes blow-outs at the skin level, which are situated over the incompetent perforators. In this case there is a blow-out over the Boyd and Dodd perforator. These protrusions are called Dow's sign.

46

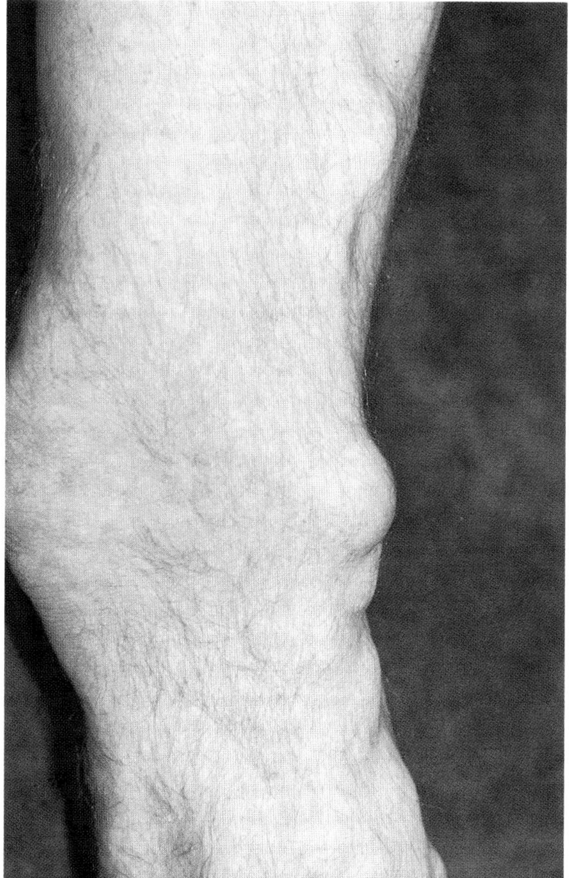

47

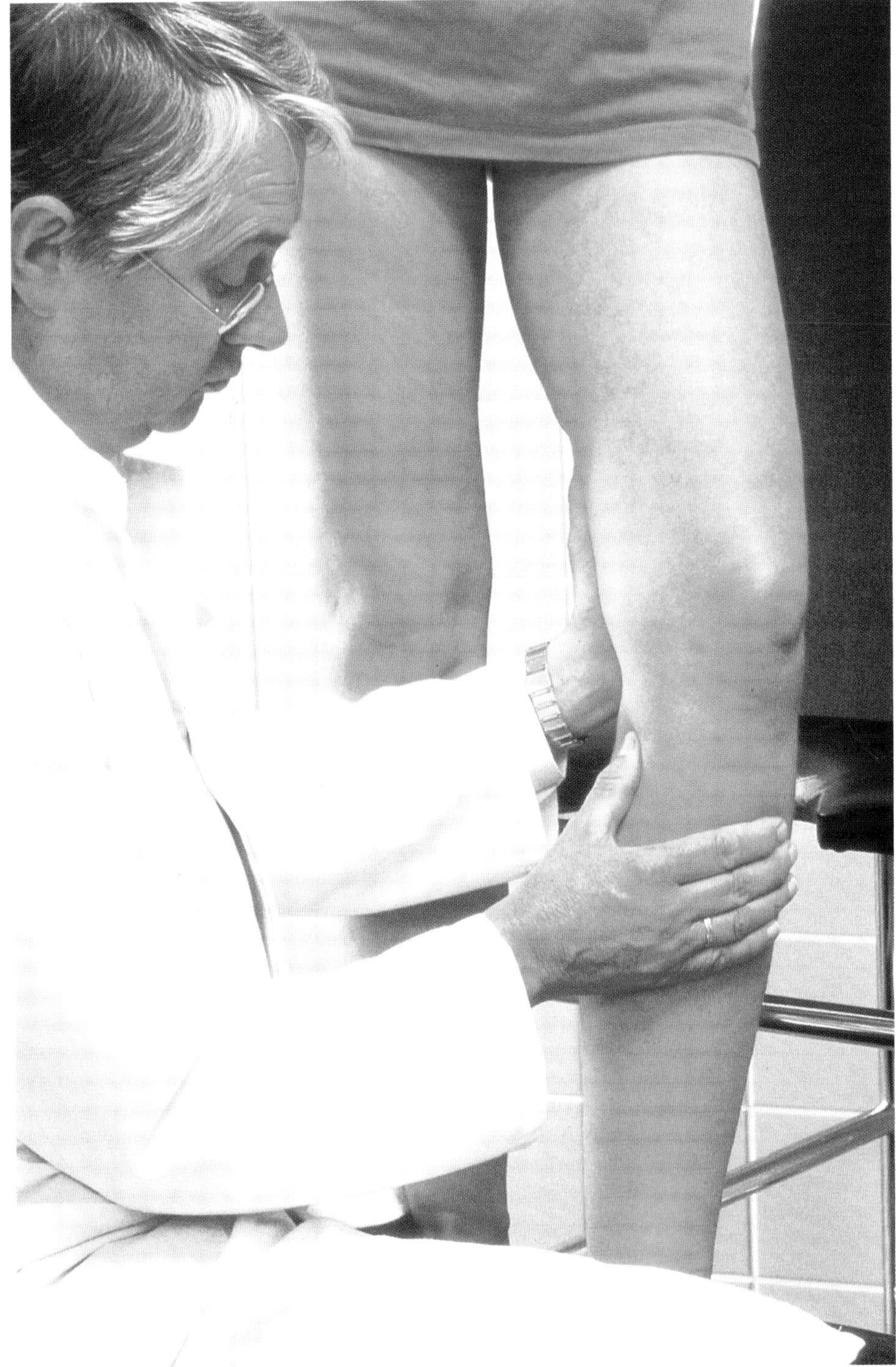

47: Incompetent perforator veins do not always cause a dramatic blow-out. A careful search for fascial defects with possible palpable veins is an important part of a phlebological examination.

48

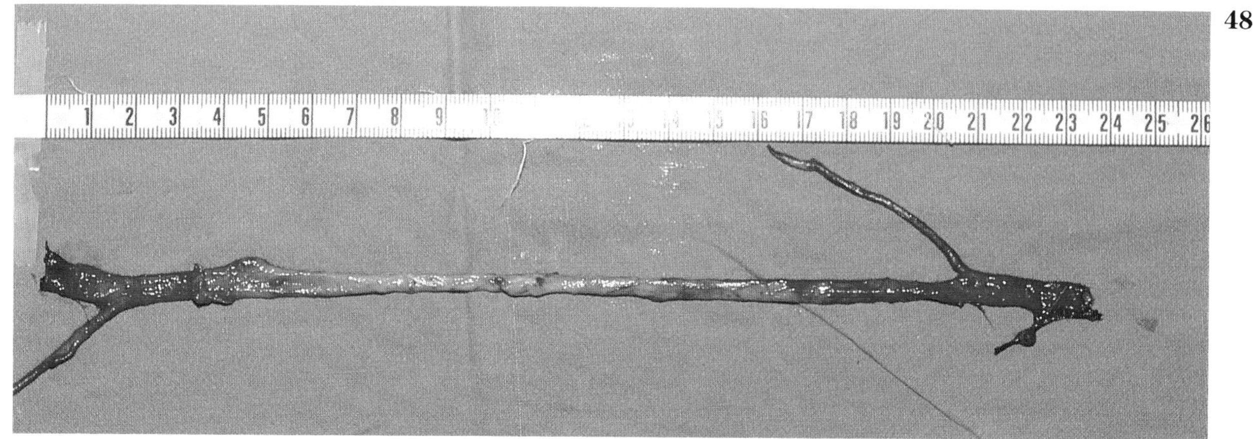

49

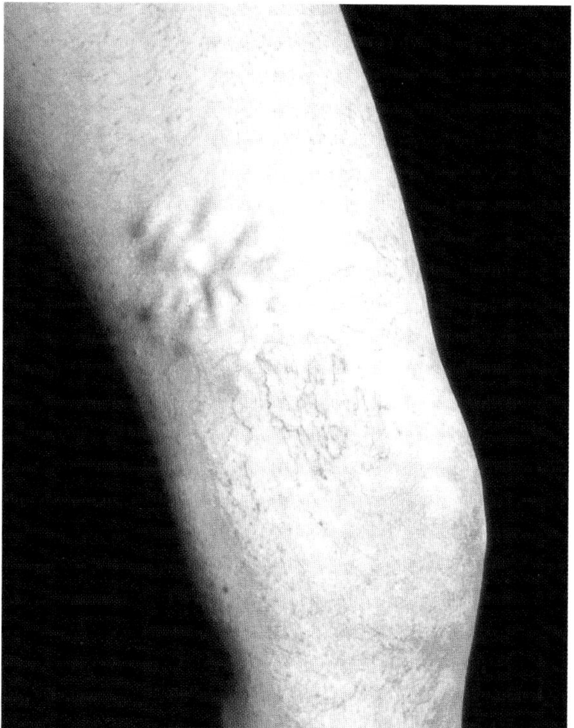

50

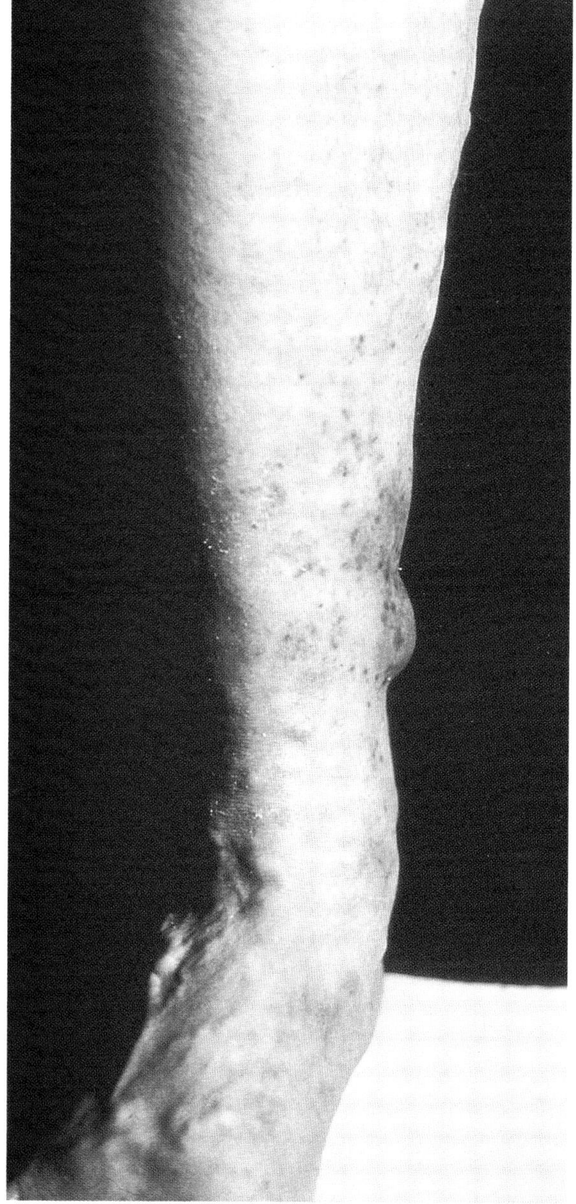

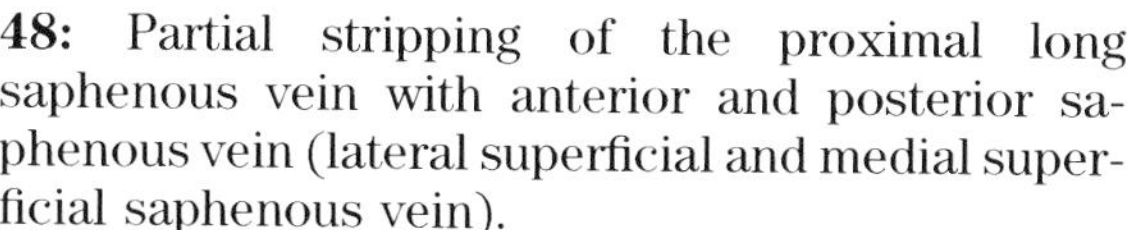

48: Partial stripping of the proximal long saphenous vein with anterior and posterior saphenous vein (lateral superficial and medial superficial saphenous vein).

49: Isolated varicosis of a Dodd perforator. The marked local venous hypertension has caused intradermal venectasias in the form of so-called spider veins.

50: Clearly visible blow-out over an incompetent so-called Cockett III perforator vein with hyperpigmentation indicating chronic venous stasis.

51

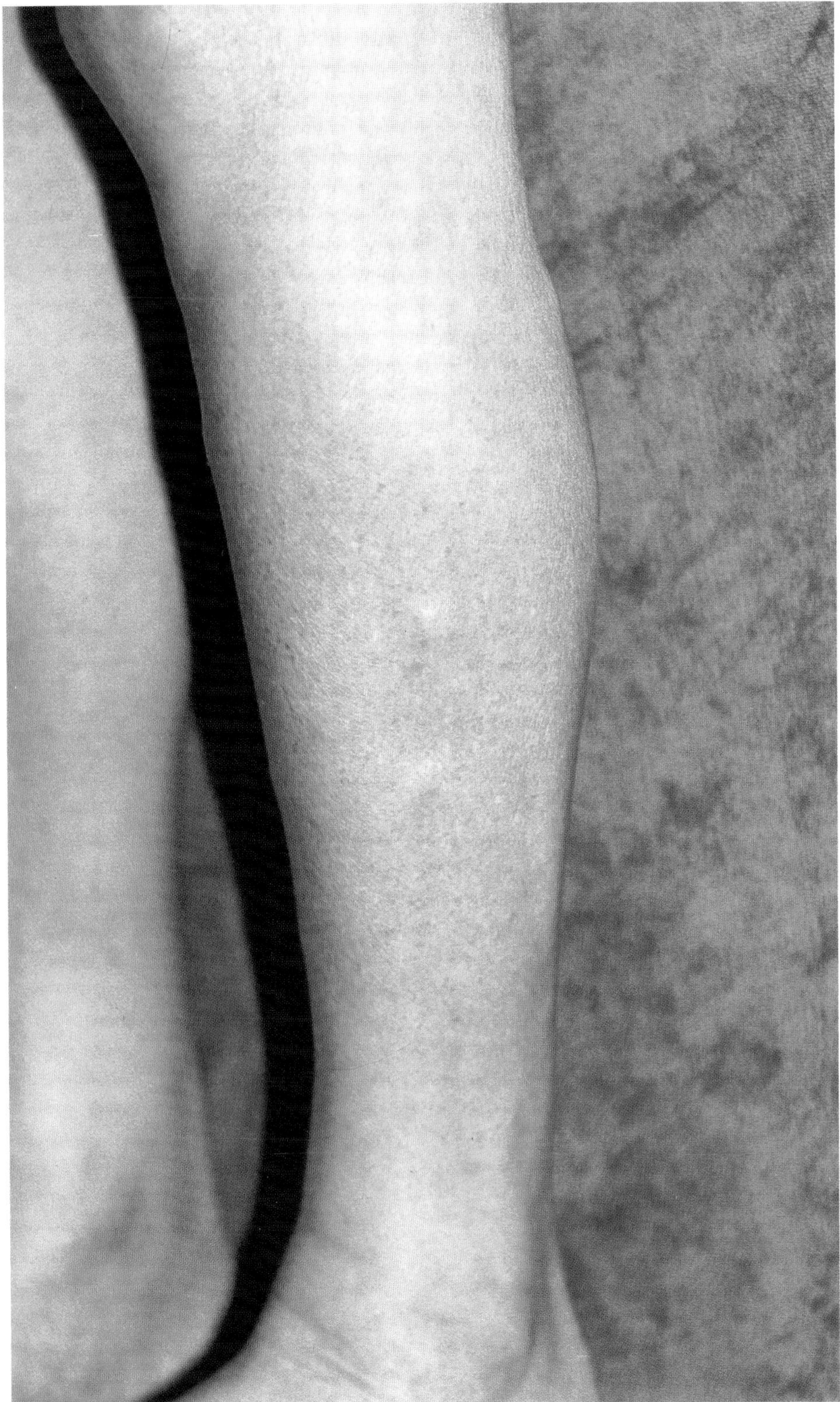

51: A venous blow-out can be mimicked by small lipomas, or by muscle hernias through fascial defects as shown in this photograph. Careful palpation and, if necessary, Doppler-demonstrated absence of flow phenomenona allow a clear differentiation from Dow's sign.

52

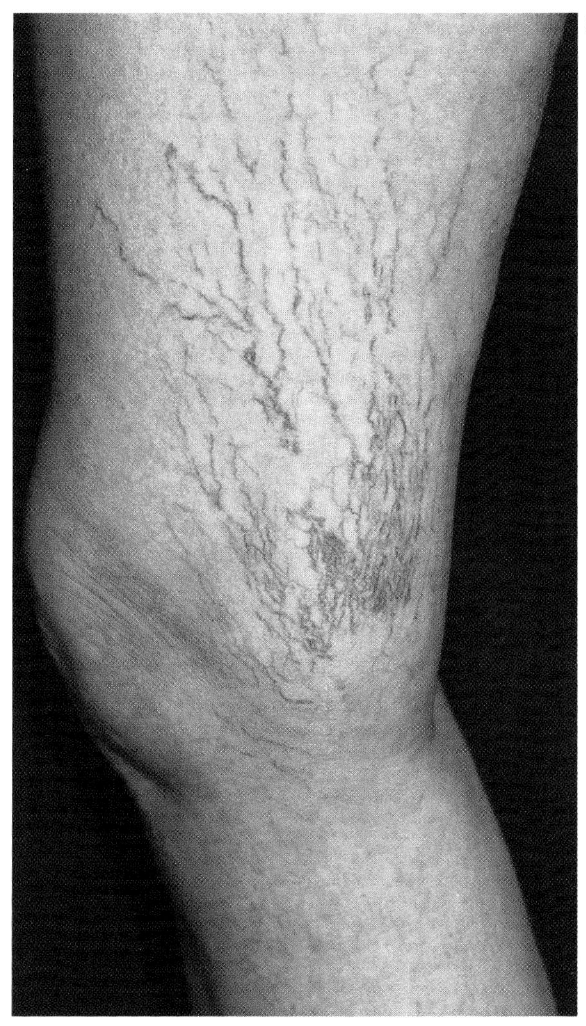

52: Spider veins are intradermal ectasias of the smallest skin veins which branch out from a feeder vein in a star-like or fan-like fashion. They have no importance for the venous haemodynamics and they do not lead to trophic skin disturbances. Not infrequently, however, they are, in the absence of other symptoms, the first indication of a dysfunction at the level of the large veins.

53

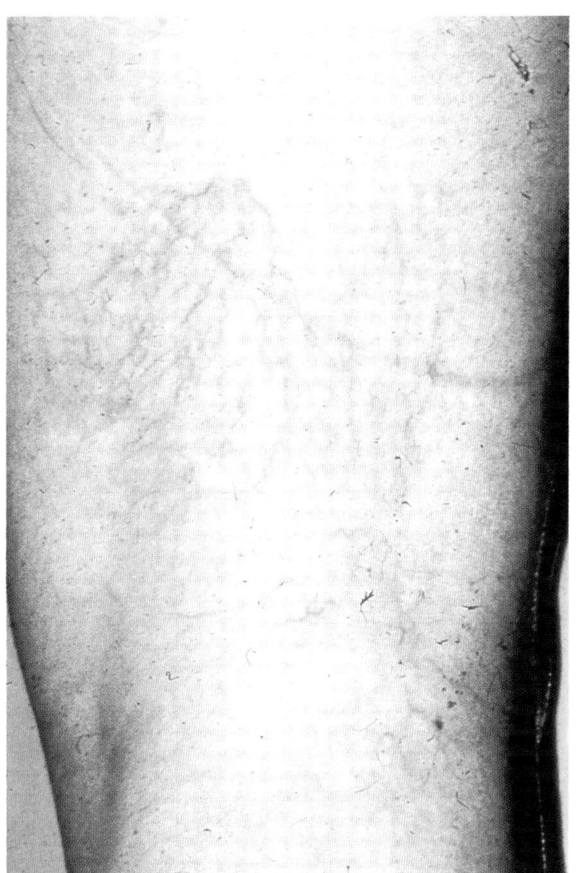

53: The combination of spider veins and varicose reticular veins is not uncommon. Many female patients experience more distress in the premenstrual period.

54

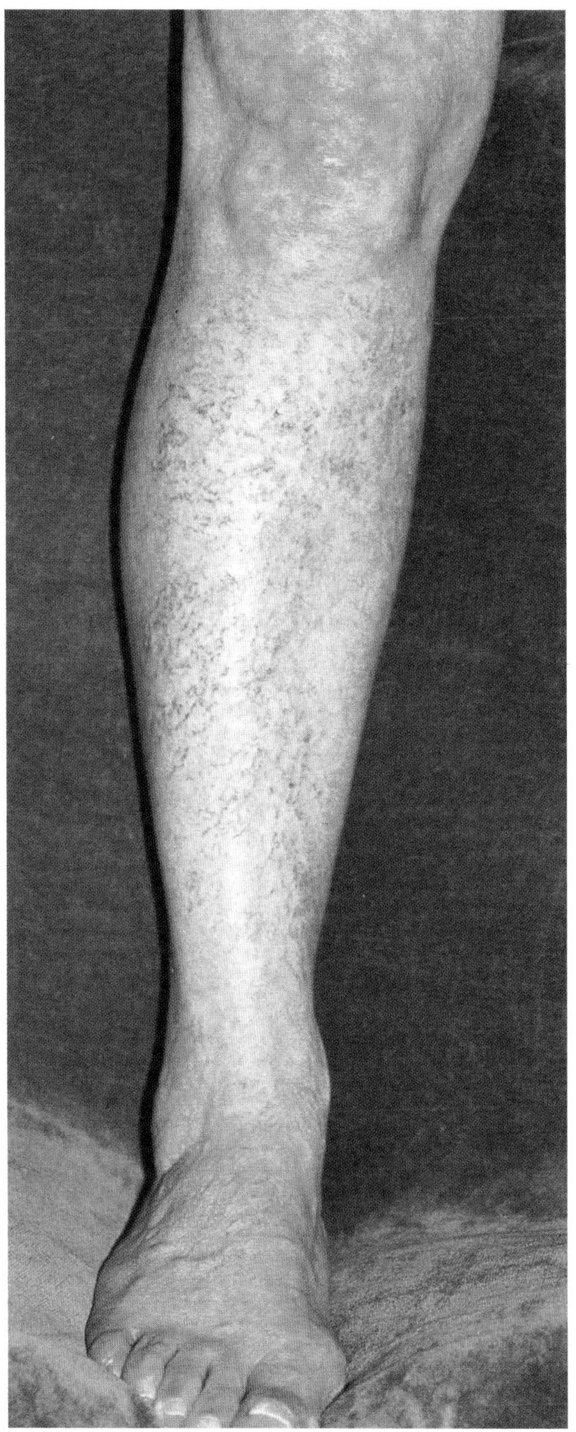

55

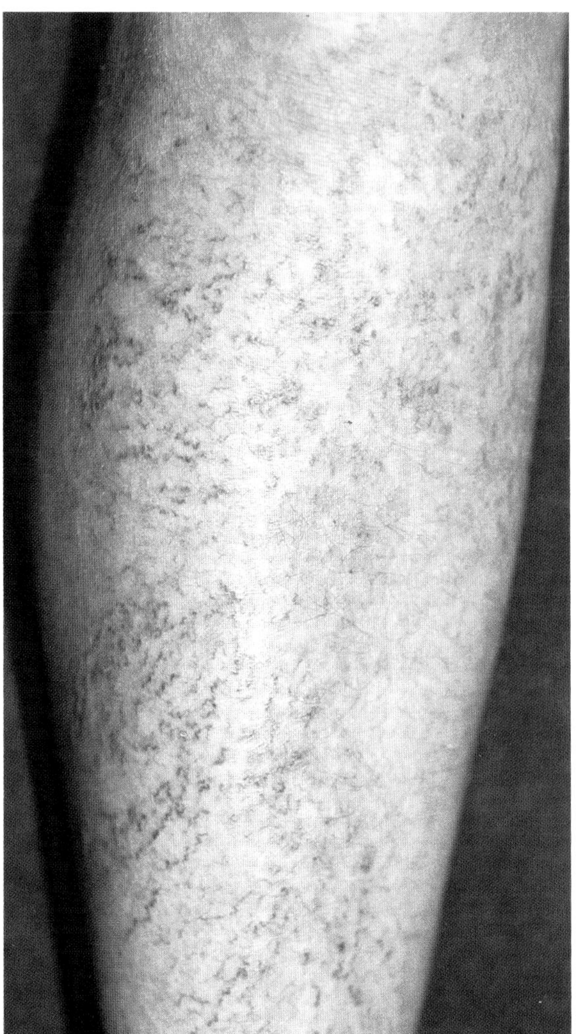

55: Reticular varicosities sometimes thrombose spontaneously, but they can also rupture, causing large subcutaneous haematomas or marked external bleeding. Sclerotherapy is indicated.

54: Varicose reticular veins are web-like, bluish venectasias at the border of cutis and subcutis. Haemodynamically they do not play an important role in the formation of a chronic venous insufficiency. However, they are often experienced as cosmetically disturbing and, in contrast to spider veins, can also lead to definitive subjective discomfort.

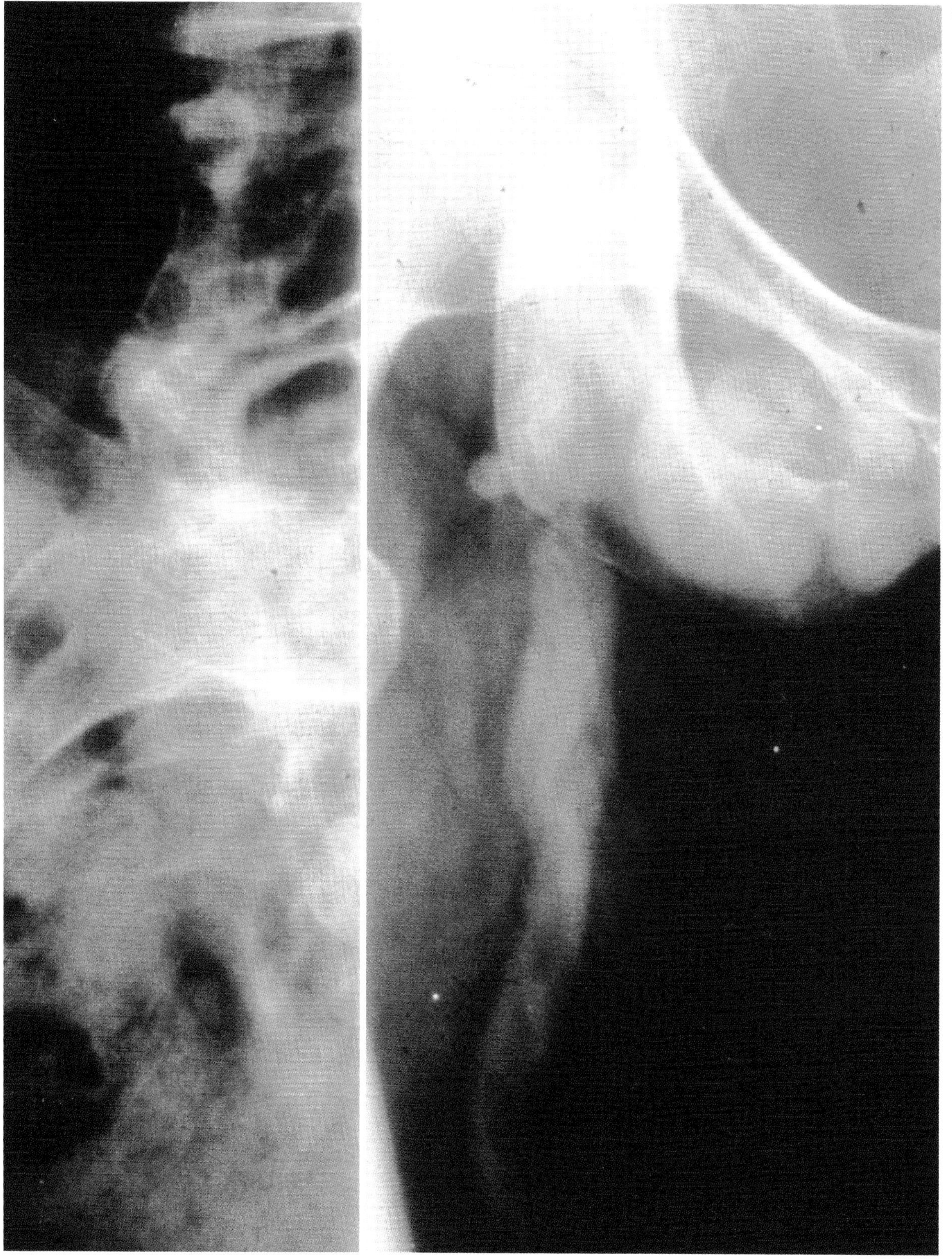

56

56: A total occlusion of the iliac vein was followed by the formation of a collateral to the opposite side. This venogram shows the collateral circulation, which could be called 'a spontaneous Palma operation'.

57

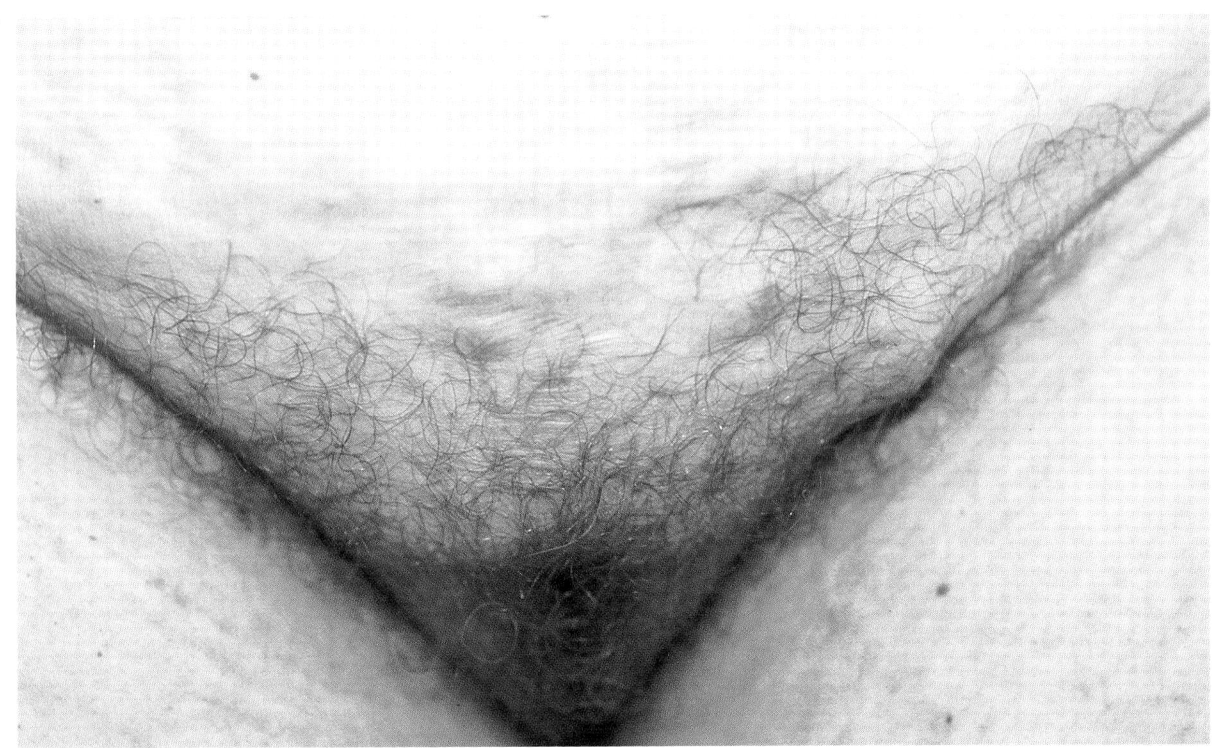

57: Suprapubic varices are secondary venectasias and represent a venous collateral circulation in the presence of a unilateral occlusion of the venous outflow pathways of the pelvis.

58

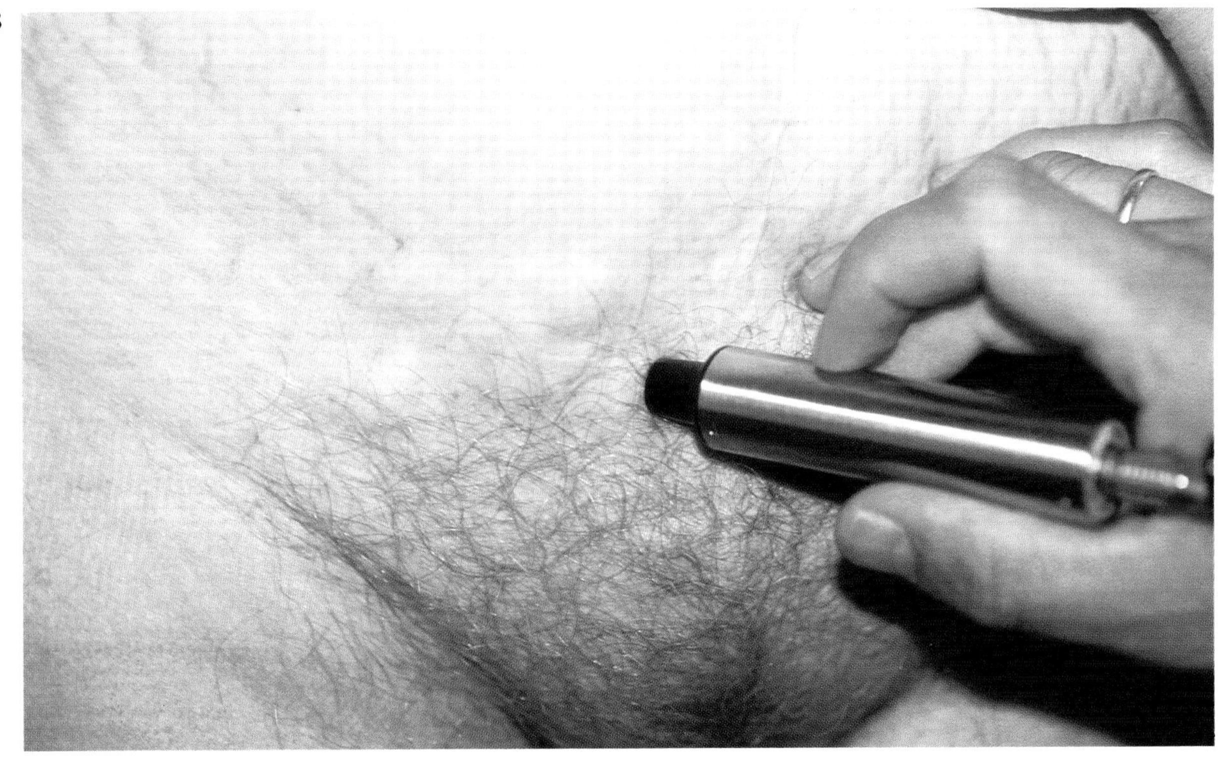

58: A Doppler-demonstrable flow in a collateral vein indicates that a haemodynamically significant alternate pathway for the pelvic venous outflow has been created.

59

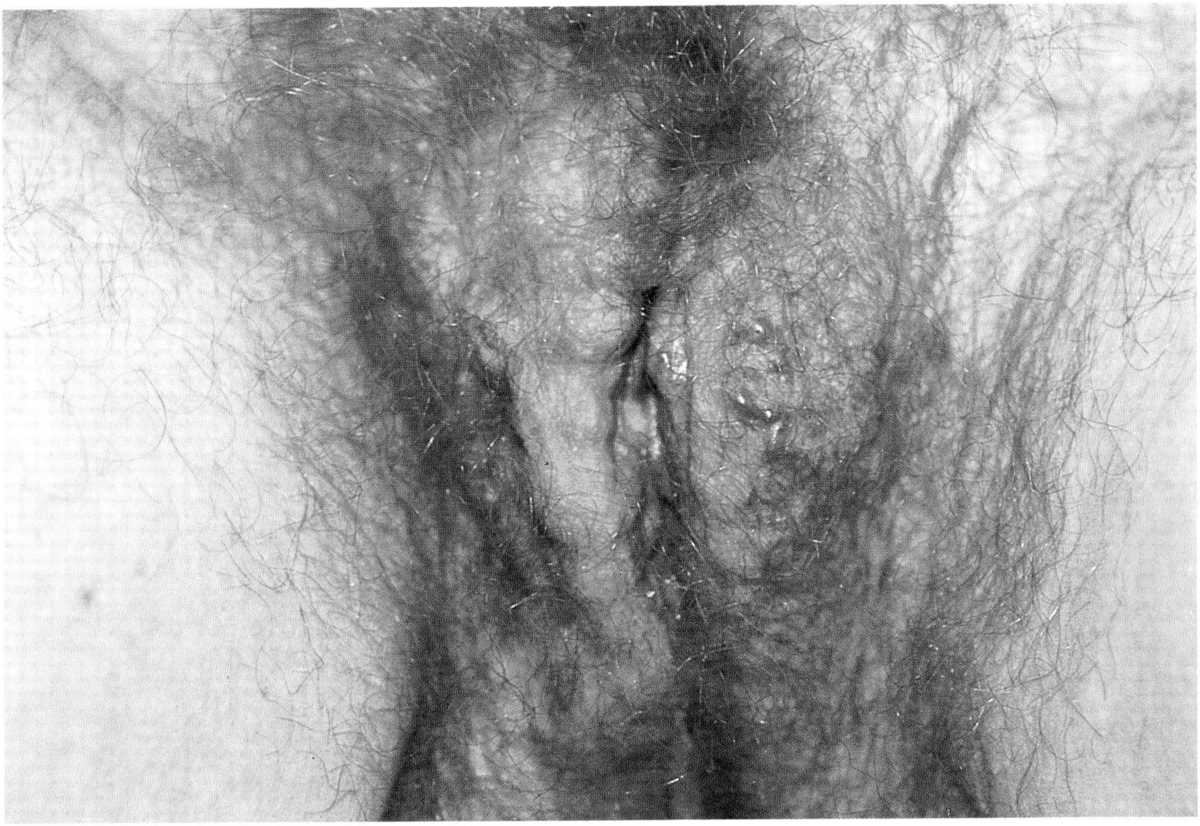

59: Vulvar varices usually occur towards the end of a pregnancy as a result of an elevated oestrogen level and increased intrapelvic pressure. They can show spontaneous regression a few weeks postpartum, which can be totally painless or be accompanied by extreme pain. One should hesitate to use sclerotherapy in these cases.

60

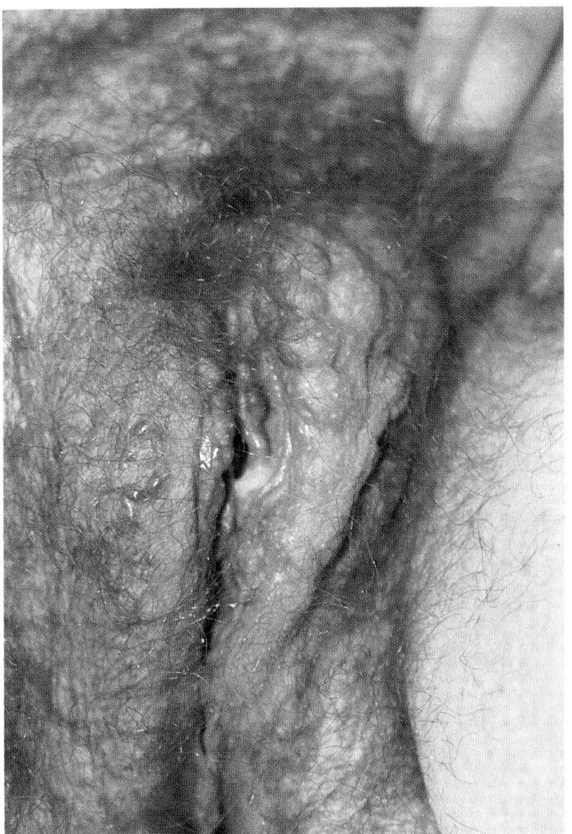

60: However, if the vulvar varices are as large as in this patient, there is a true indication for sclerotherapy, because a rupture could cause a life-threatening bleeding. After the sclerotherapy a special compression stocking is necessary.

61

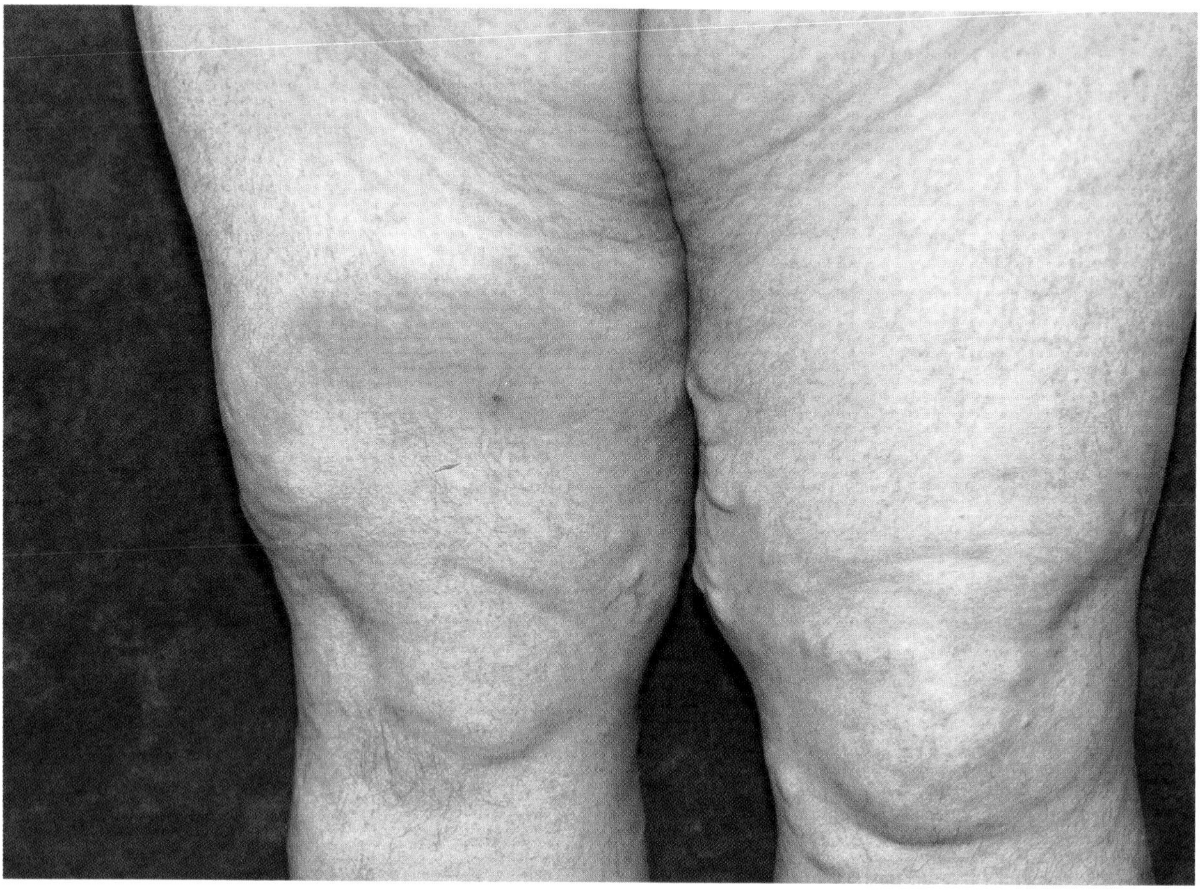

62

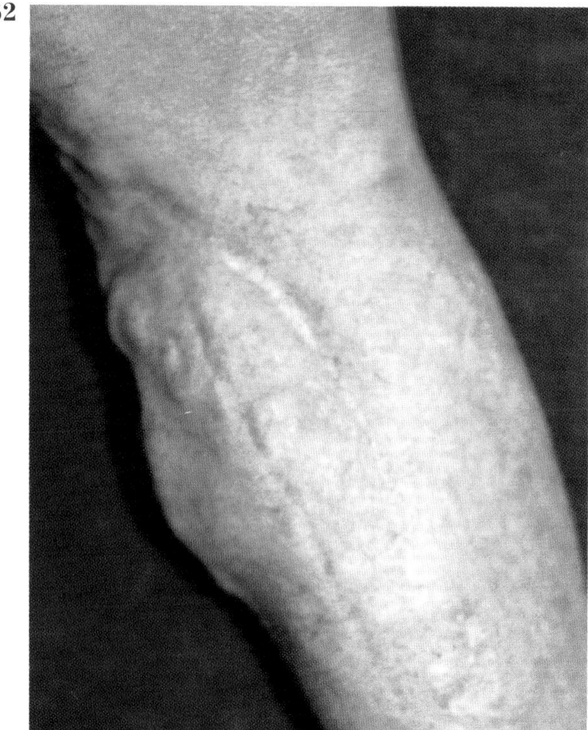

61: In this female patient, an inadequate varicose vein operation led to a recurrence of the varicosis. The surgical incision is too far distal for a ligation and division, and as a result the noninterrupted tributaries at the junction lead the reflux more distally.

62: A recurrence followed a Rindfleisch operation, which is no longer used. In this operation the long saphenous vein in the area to be treated was completely dissected and removed *in toto*.

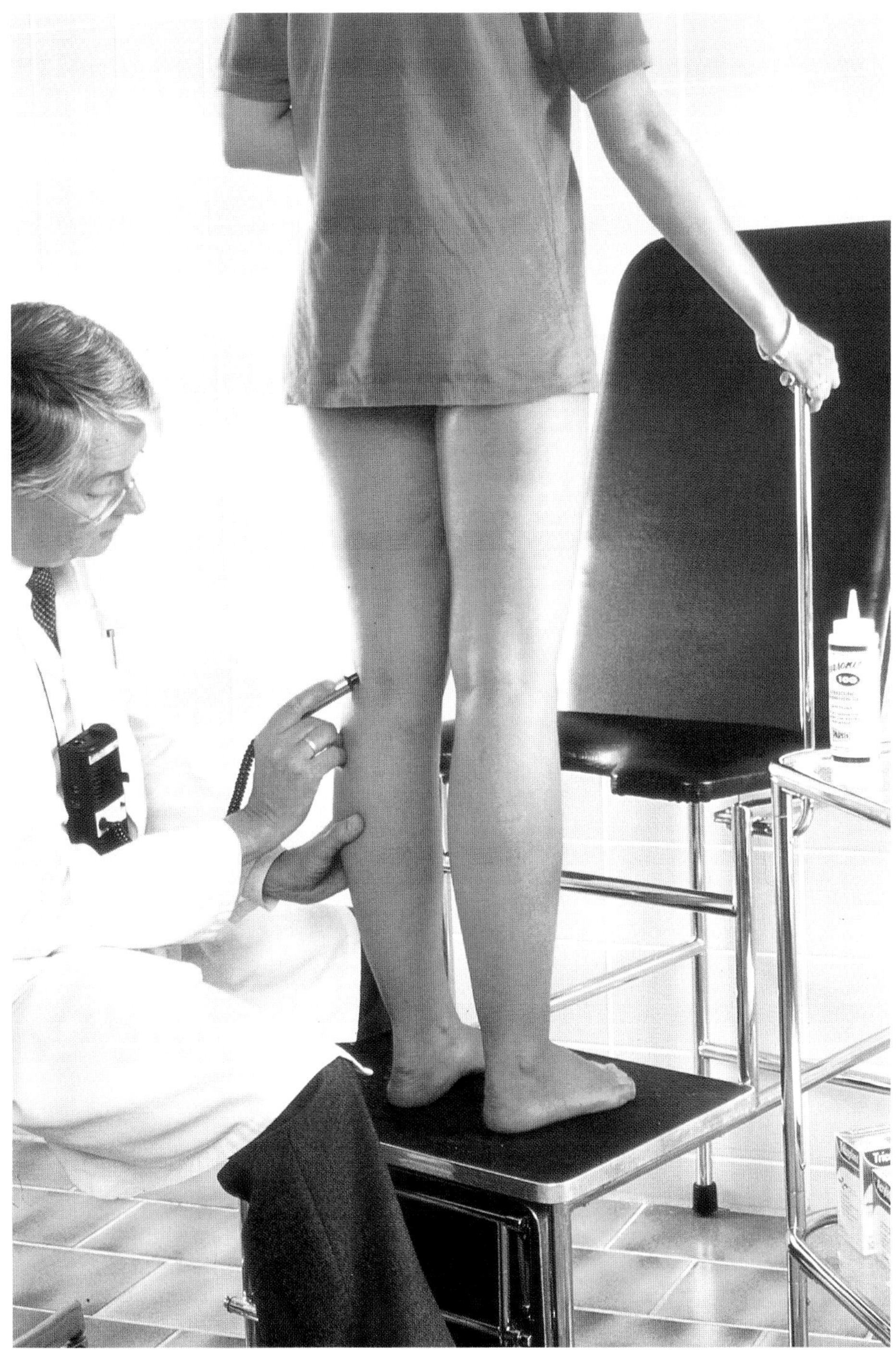

63: A unidirectional Doppler examination can show an abnormal flow reversal of venous blood. A Valsalva manoeuvre or a compression and decompression manoeuvre proximal and distal to the area examined can show a venous reflux, indicating a malfunctioning of the venous valves. There are no normal respiratory fluctuations of venous flow over an area of acute thrombosis. Proximal to the occlusion the augmentation normally caused by distal compression is absent. A high-frequency venous flow without respiratory fluctuations can also be heard over collateral veins or partially blocked vein segments.

64

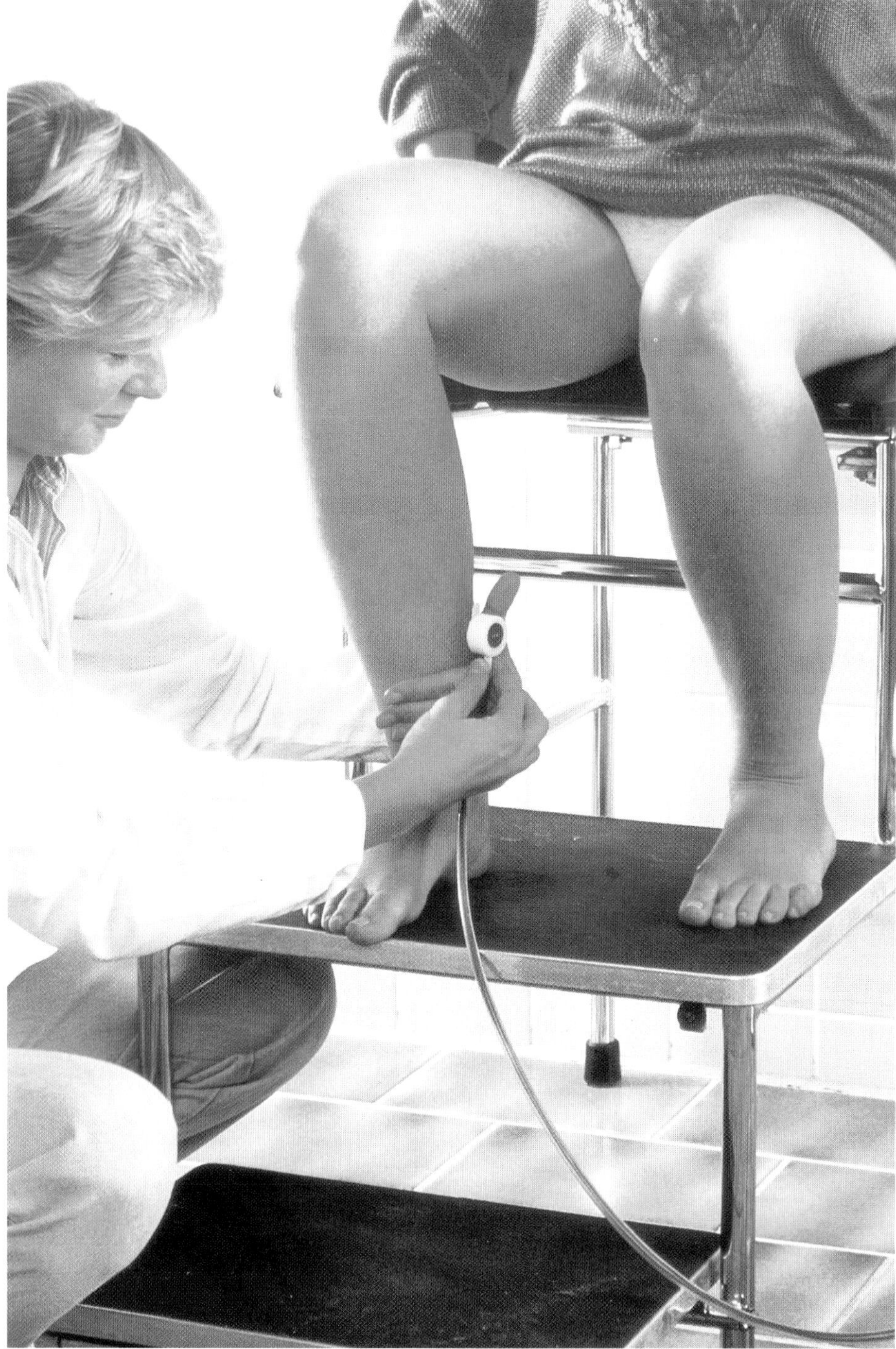

64: With light-reflection-rheography (LRR) or photoplethysmography (PPG) the venous haemodynamics of the skin can be assessed. The refilling time of the cutaneous venous plexus is measured after a defined amount of exercise. The method makes it possible to draw conclusions regarding the function of the entire venous system of the leg.

65

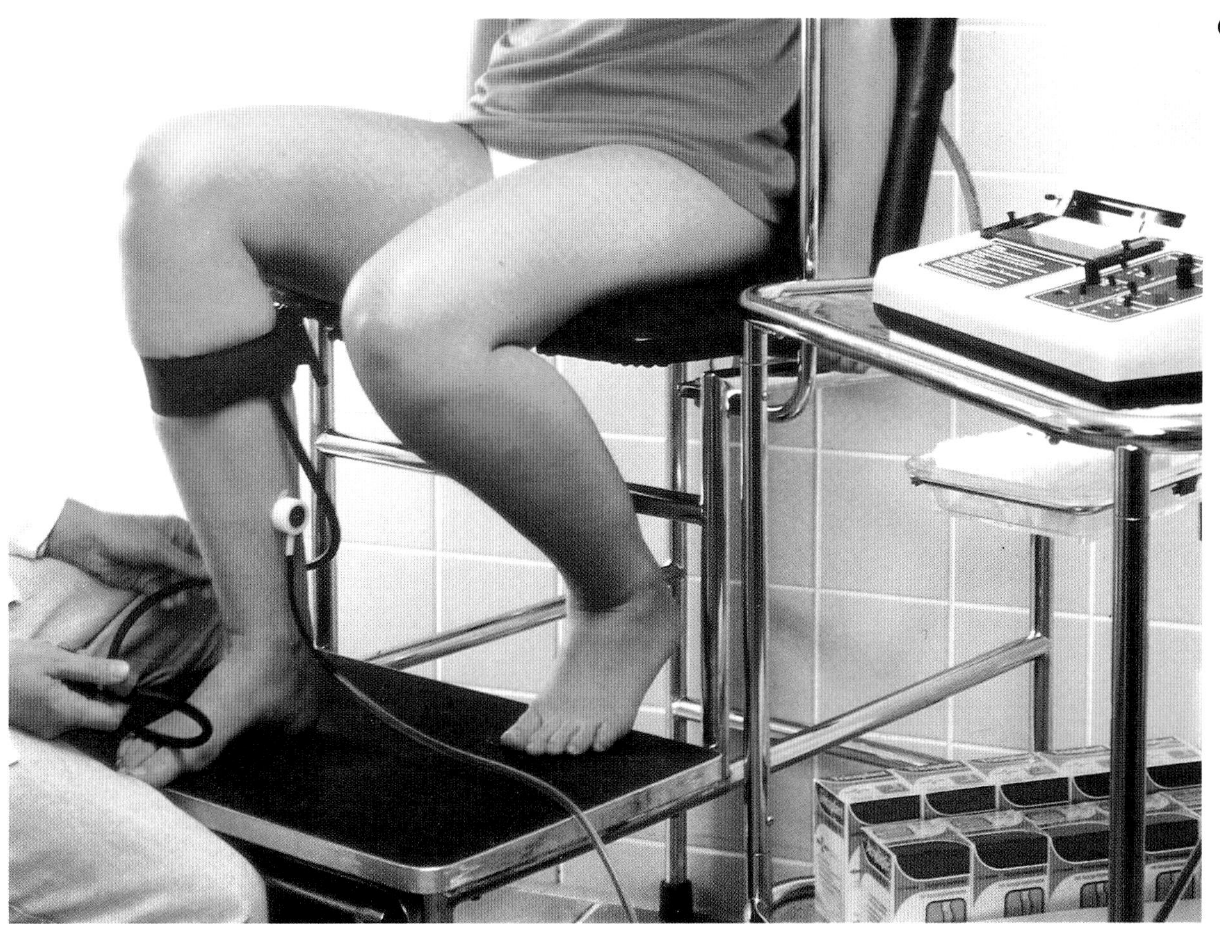

65: By compressing the superficial veins with a tourniquet, the improvement of the venous return by operative methods, sclerosis or compression therapy can be predicted.

66 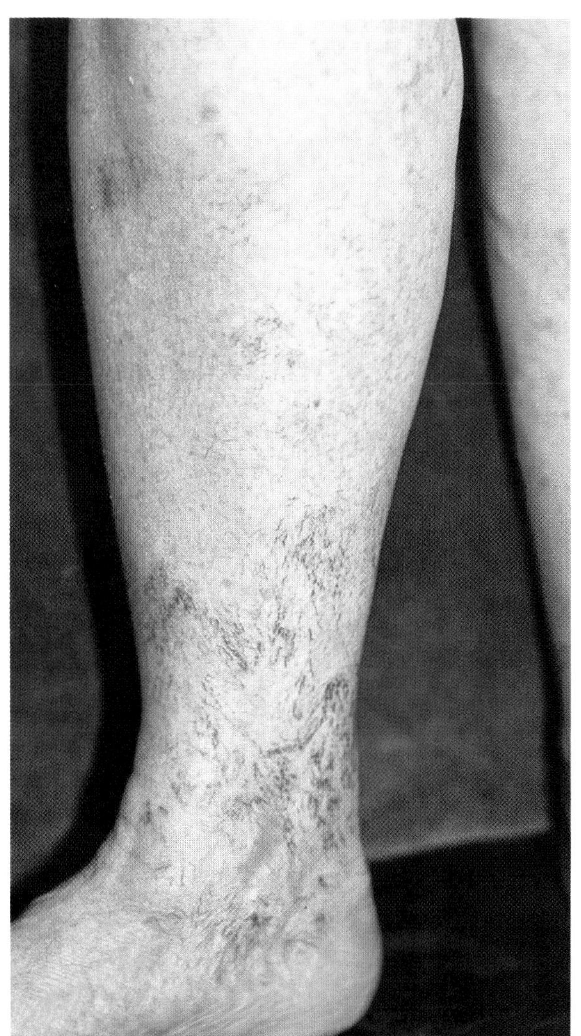

Chronic venous insufficiency (CVI)

A chronic dysfunction in the superficial or deep venous system leads to venous hypertension. When the failing ability of the venous system to transport the blood can no longer be compensated by the lymphatic system, trophic tissue abnormalities as a sign of chronic venous insufficiency (CVI) manifest themselves. According to the skin changes, three stages can be recognized:

Stage I
Corona phlebectatica paraplantaris.

Stage II
Trophic skin changes (siderosclerosis, hyperpigmentation, depigmentation, stasis dermatitis).

Stage III
Active or healed stasis ulcer.

66: The corona phlebectatica paraplantaris should be differentiated from spider veins in the distal lower leg.

67: The first clear sign of chronic venous stasis is the corona phlebectatica paraplantaris. It consists of 6–8 venectasias in the ankle area and border of the foot (like pearls in a crown), in combination with venectasias arranged like the lines in a spider's web, and red-bluish stasis patches.

67 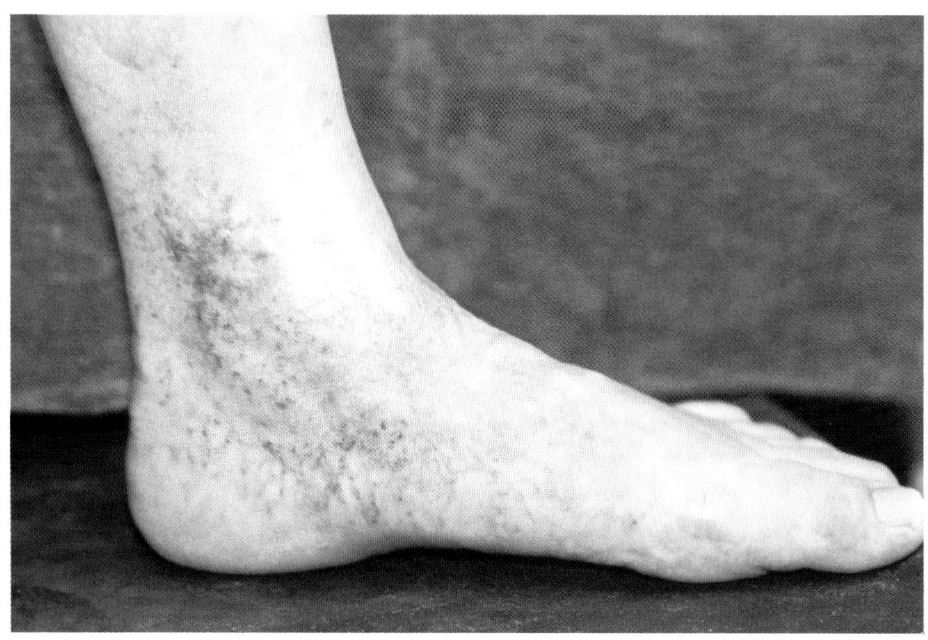

68: Stage II of CVI is characterized by pigmentation changes in the skin. The hyperpigmentations originate from small punctiform bleedings in the upper corium, which are converted into haemosiderin and stored. Porcelain-like whitish areas are typical for the depigmentation of atrophie blanche, which is the stage just before CVI Stage III. Combinations of the above occur frequently.

69: In the smooth depigmented areas of atrophie blanche, only atrophied arterials can be found. Extreme pain may be present (vasculitis alba). In these cases, in addition to the usual compression therapy, a short-term treatment with steroids is indicated.

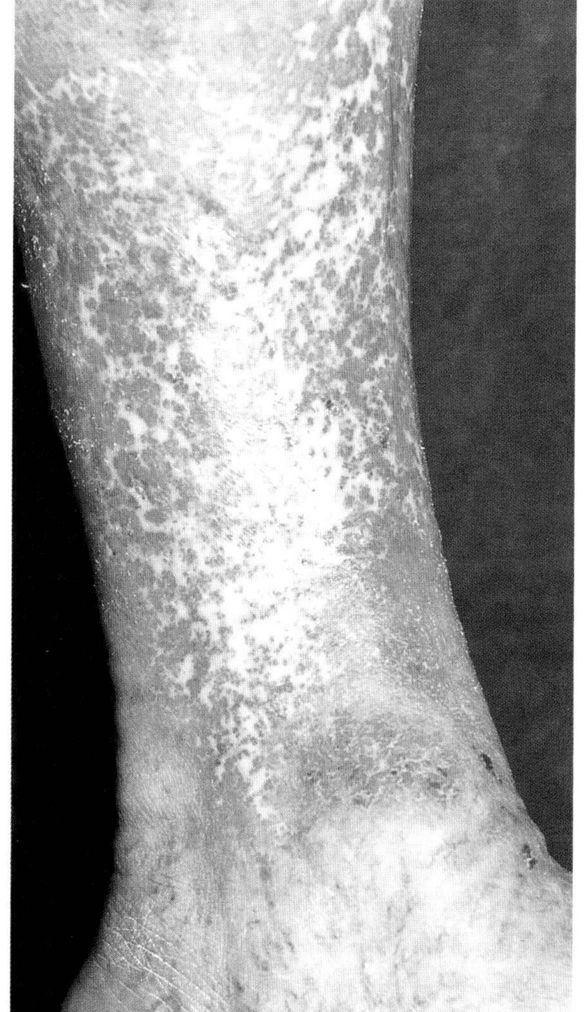

68

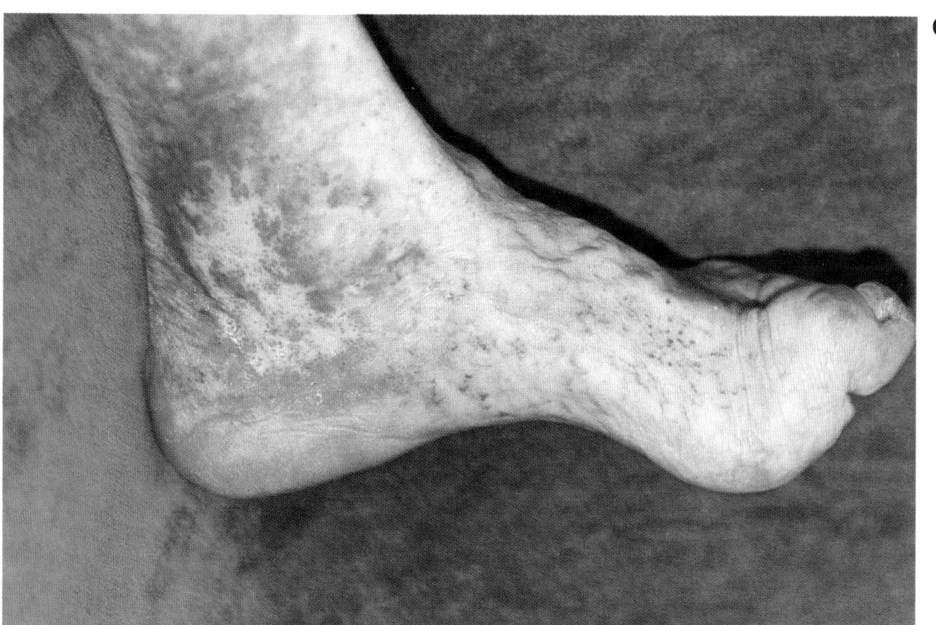

69

70

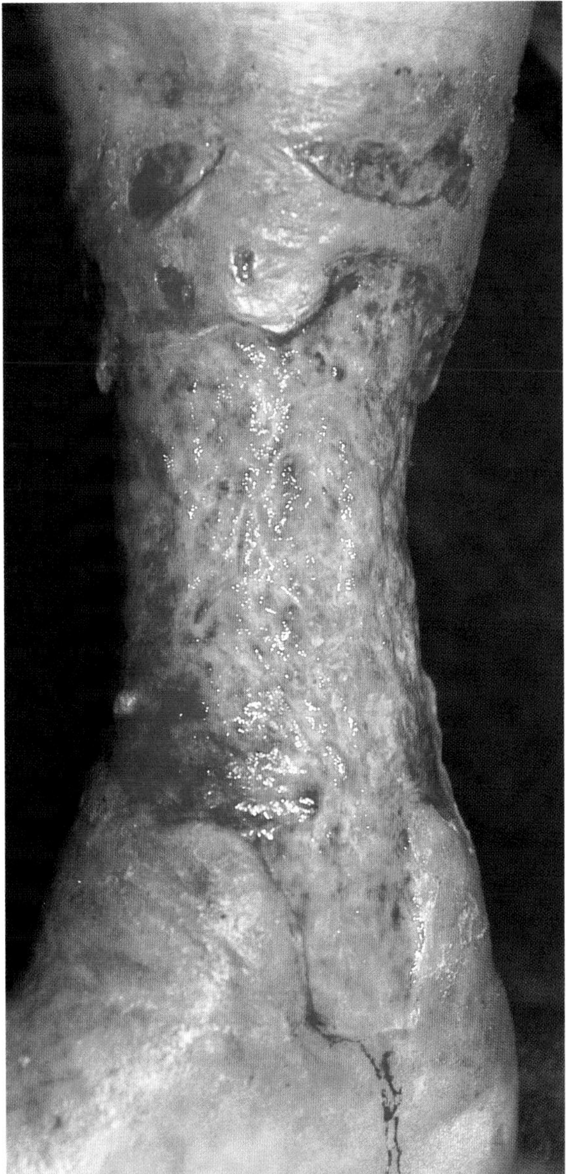

71

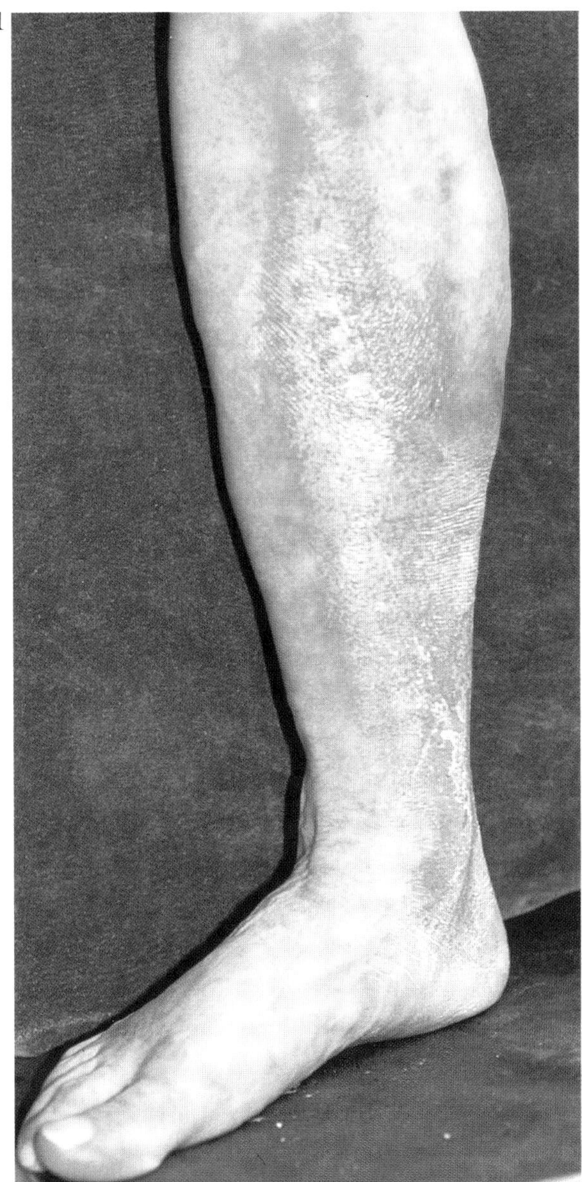

70: An active or healed venous stasis ulcer is the hallmark of Stage III of CVI. A circumferential defect of the distal lower leg is called a gaiter ulcer, in this case caused by a post-thrombotic syndrome.

71: Even extensive ulcerations can be made to heal with the proper therapy. However, the skin covering such areas will always be more vulnerable and has to be protected with continuing compression. Before any compression treatment is initiated, coexisting arterial occlusive disease with critical closure pressures has to be excluded.

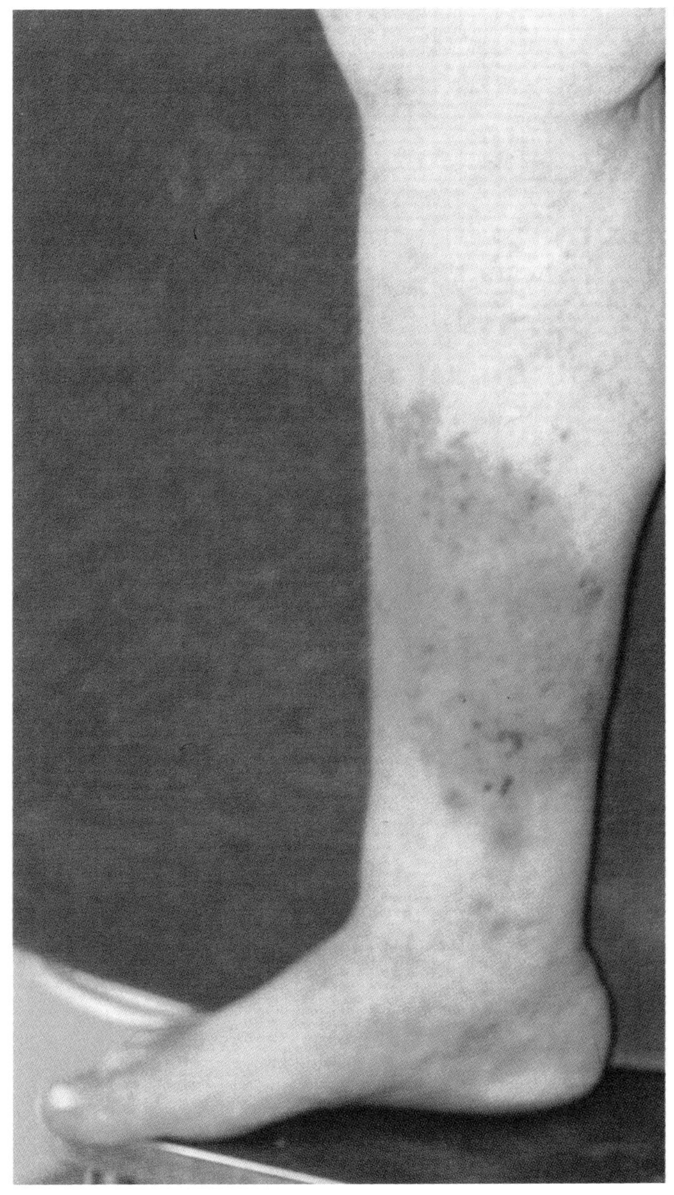

72

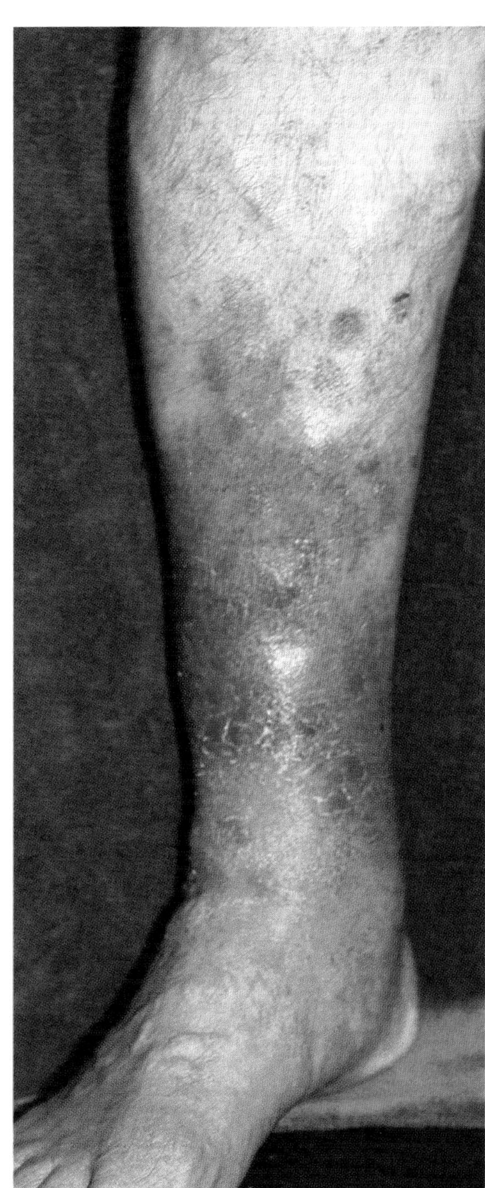

73

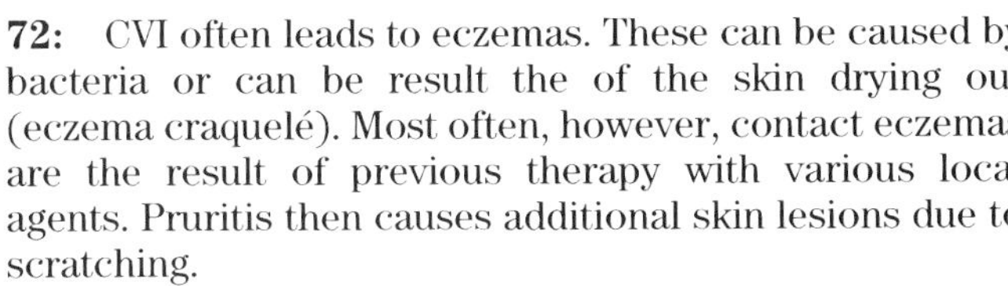

72: CVI often leads to eczemas. These can be caused by bacteria or can be result the of the skin drying out (eczema craquelé). Most often, however, contact eczemas are the result of previous therapy with various local agents. Pruritis then causes additional skin lesions due to scratching.

73: Hypodermitis shows the classical signs of inflammation (redness, increased temperature and pain). It is caused by an inflammatory reaction to the proteins which have filtered out from the intravascular compartment resulting in fibrosis of the dermis.

74

75

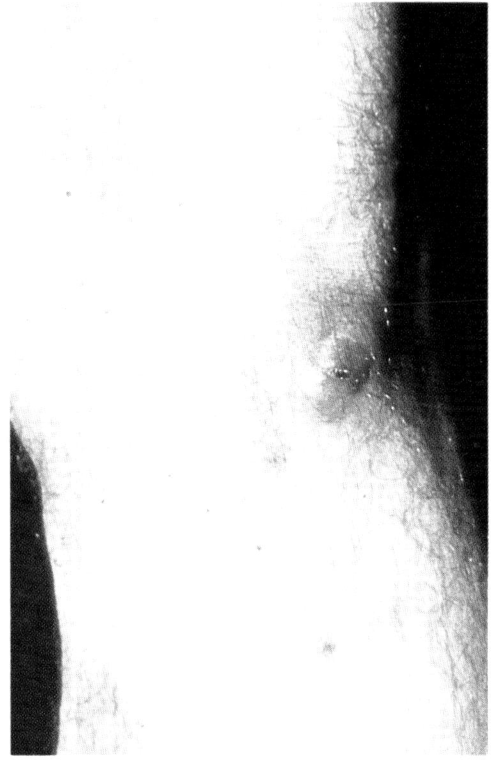

75: Inflammation of the superficial veins can occur after soft tissue trauma. It is most common, however, in veins with varicose changes.

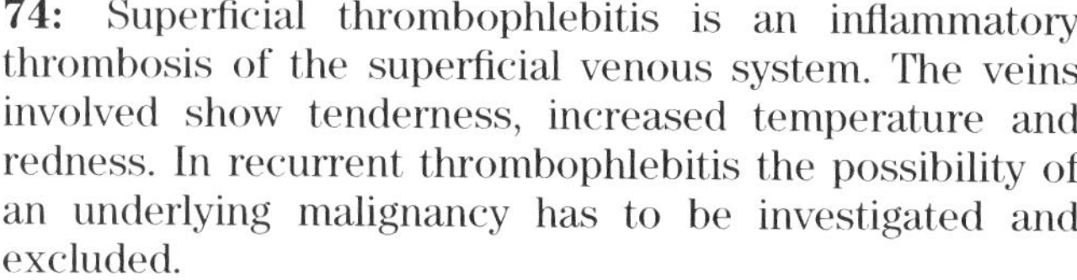

74: Superficial thrombophlebitis is an inflammatory thrombosis of the superficial venous system. The veins involved show tenderness, increased temperature and redness. In recurrent thrombophlebitis the possibility of an underlying malignancy has to be investigated and excluded.

76

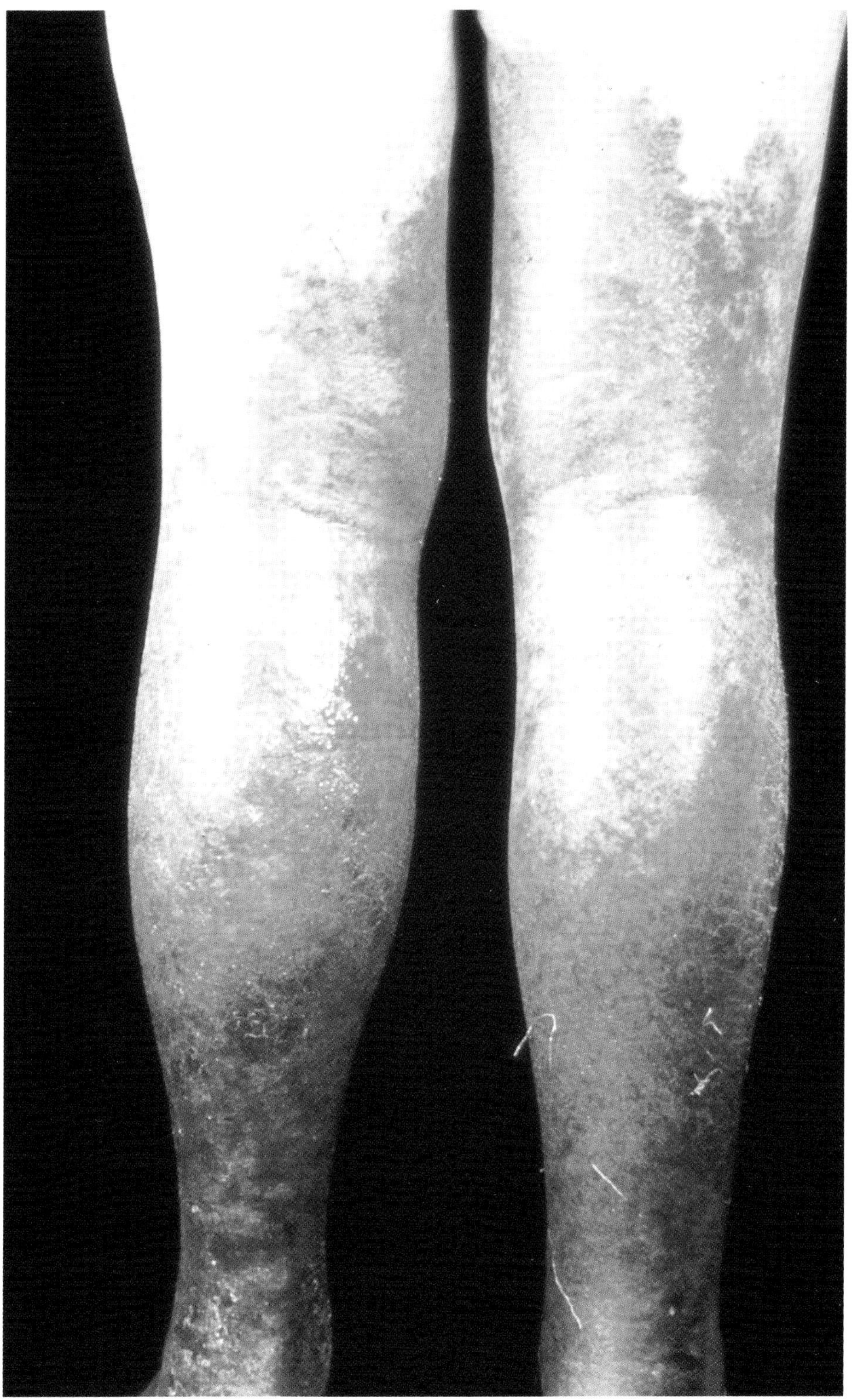

76: Thrombophlebitis is easily differentiated from erysipelas, a streptococcal infection with fever, large areas of redness and usually obvious inguinal lymphadenopathy with tenderness.

77

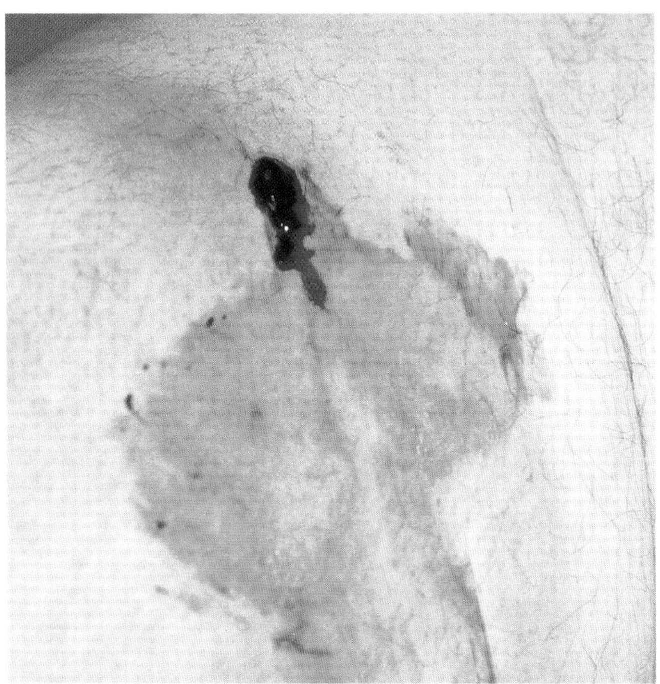

77: The patient's symptoms can be rapidly relieved by making an incision and evacuating the thrombotic material. If this method is not possible because of the age of the thrombosis or its location, adequate compression has to be used while the patient is immobilized, if necessary supplemented with systemic anti-inflammatory treatment.

78

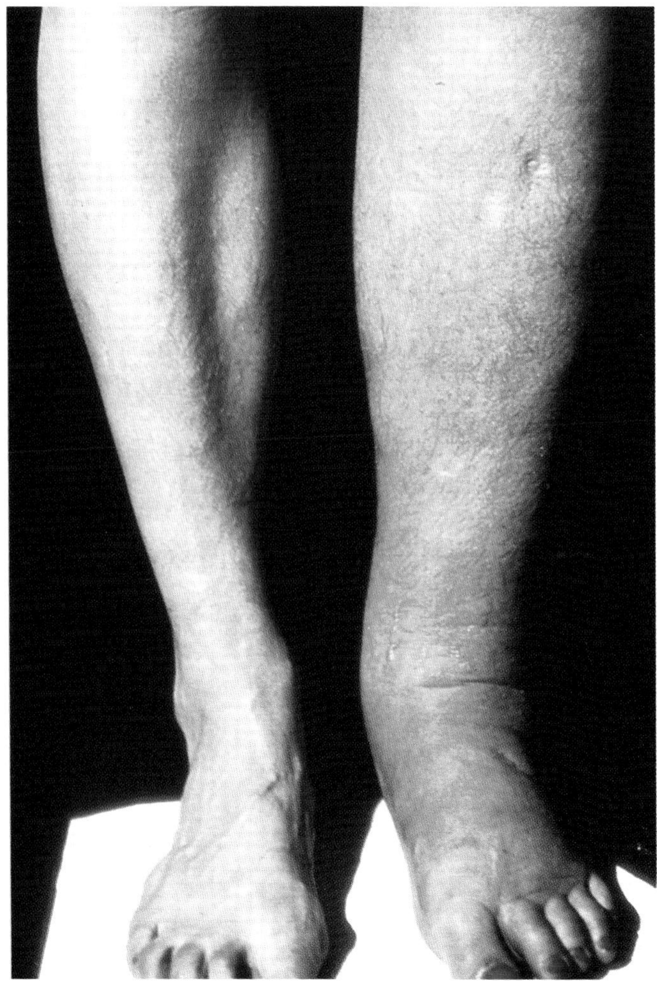

78: Phlegmasia cerulia dolens is an acute occlusion of the deep and superficial veins. It constitutes an angiological emergency because of the high rate of embolism and the impairment of the arterial inflow by the rapidly developing oedema. The patient is further endangered because of the shock syndrome. Apart from the marked oedema, the skin is livid and cool and there is severe pain in the extremity.

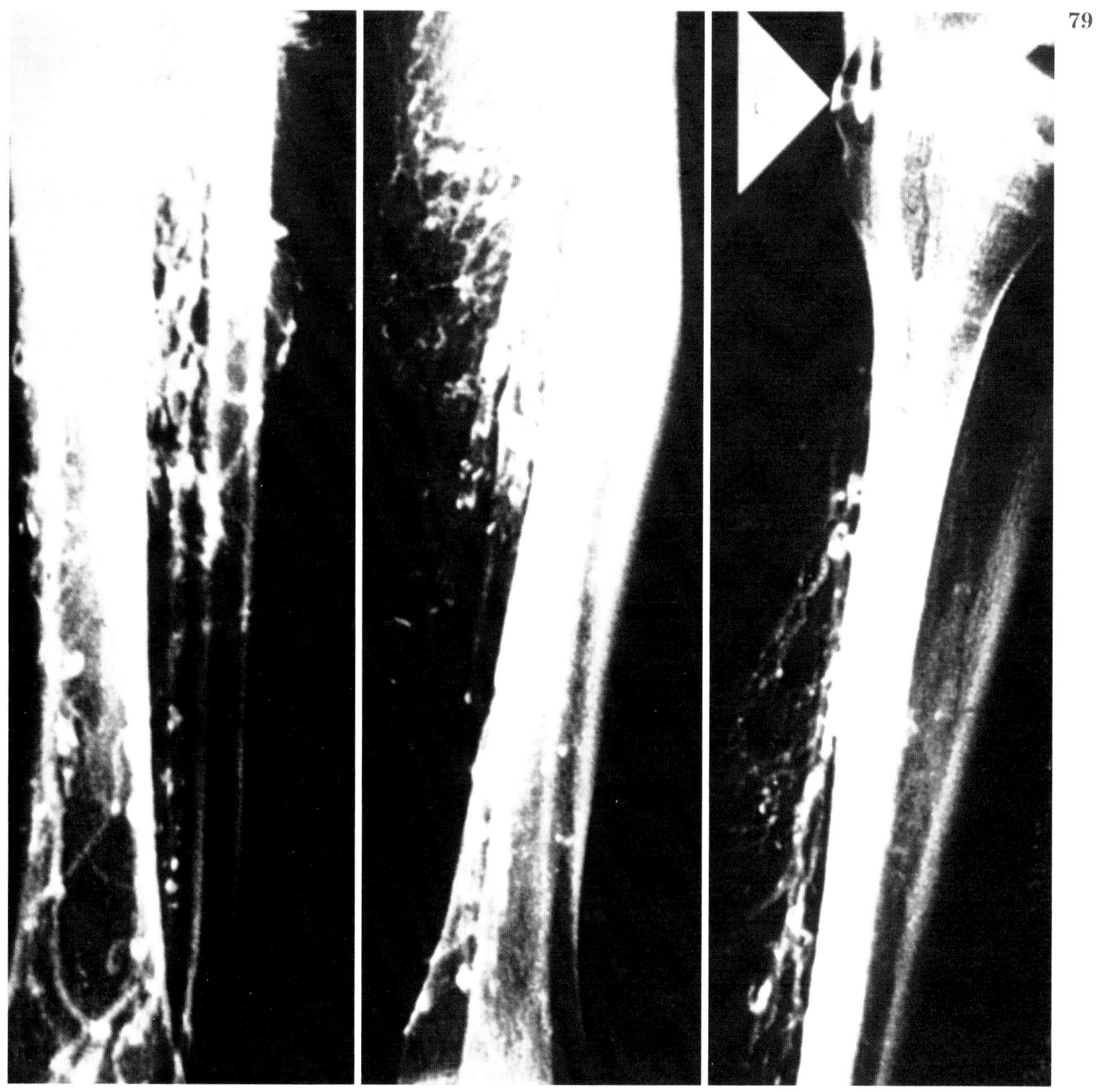

79

79: Venogram showing extensive lower leg thrombosis. The arrow indicates the tail of the thrombus.

80

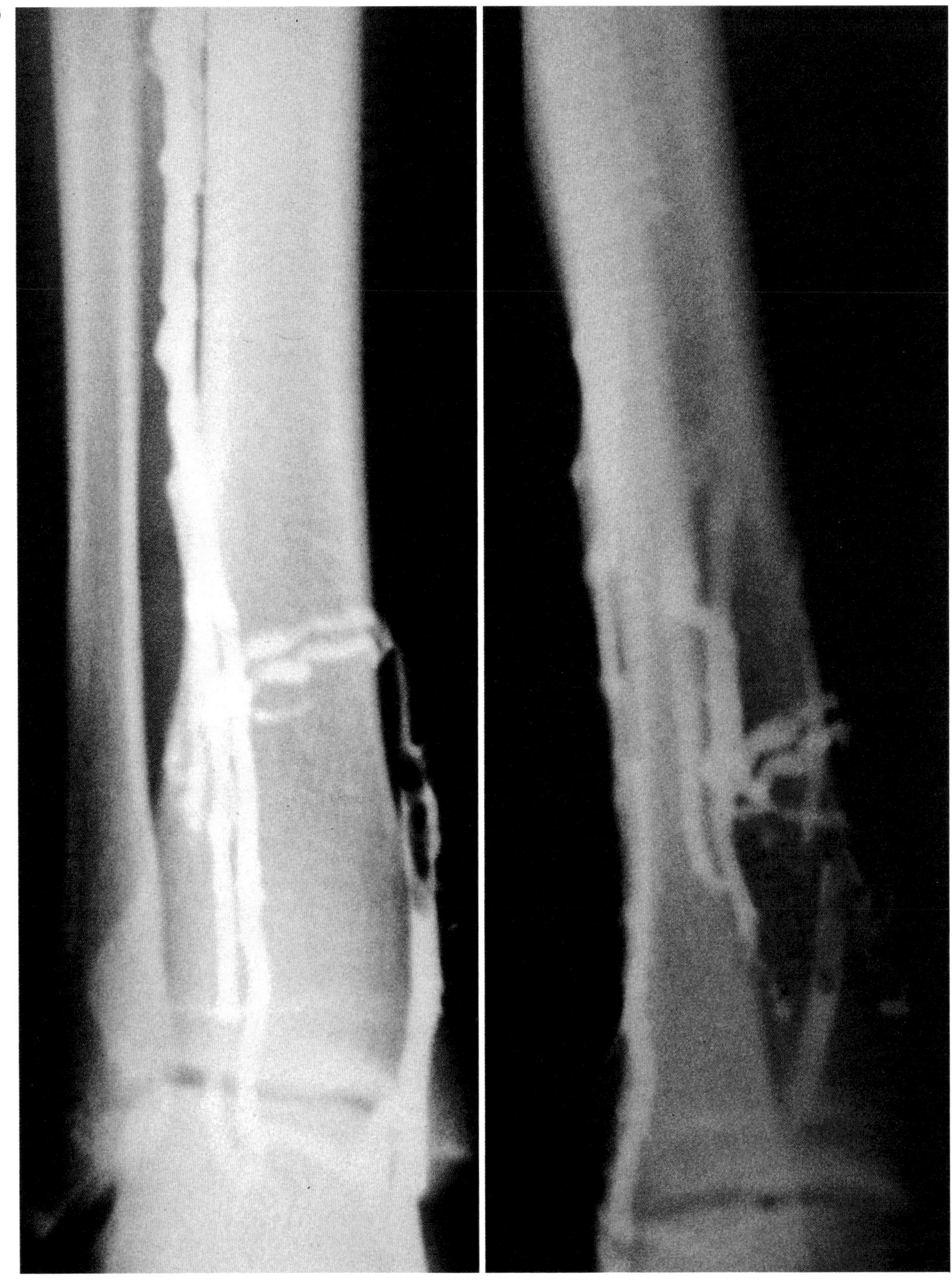

80: Thrombotic occlusion of the posterior tibial vein.

81

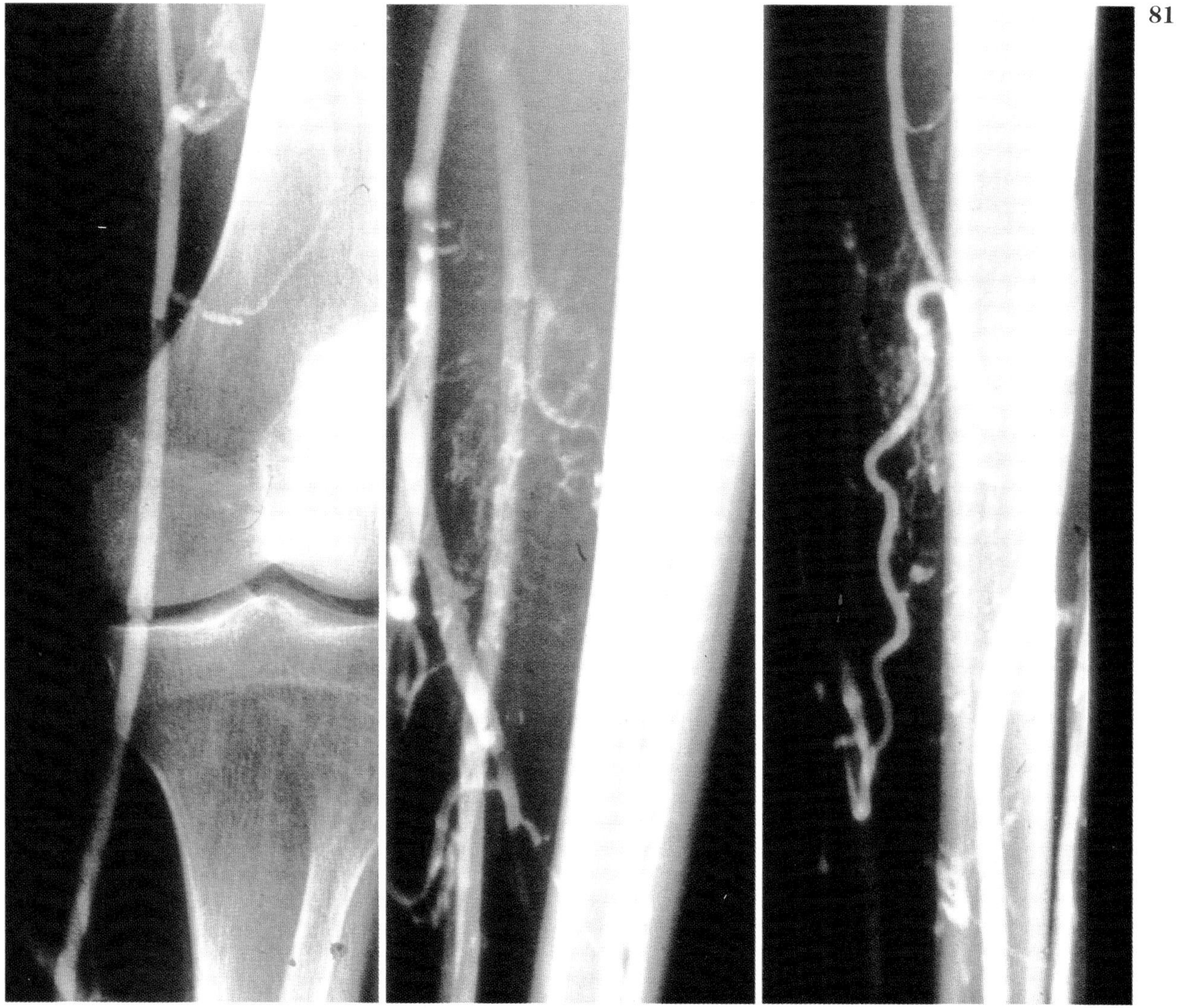

81: The superficial femoral vein is completely occluded by a fresh thrombus. No contrast material can be seen around the thrombus.

82

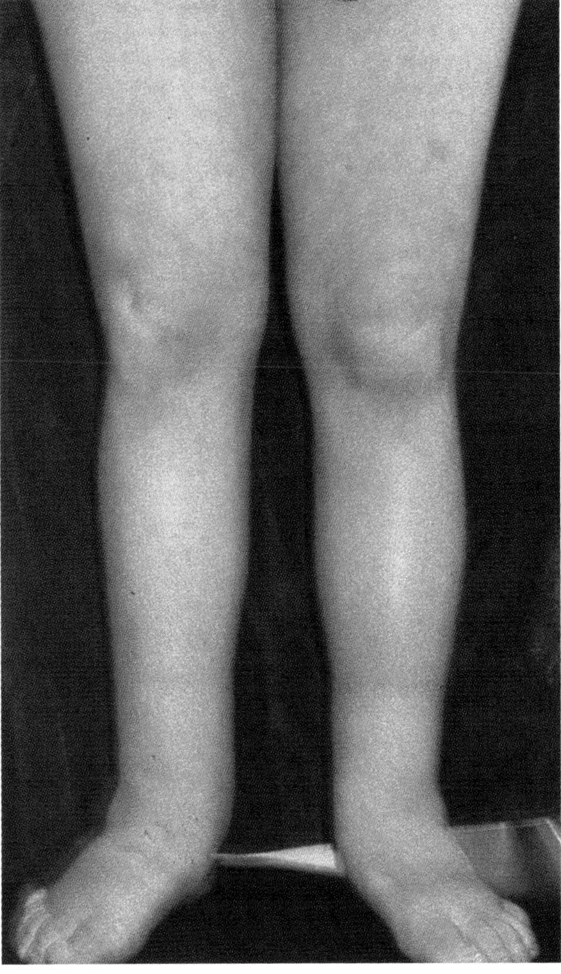

84

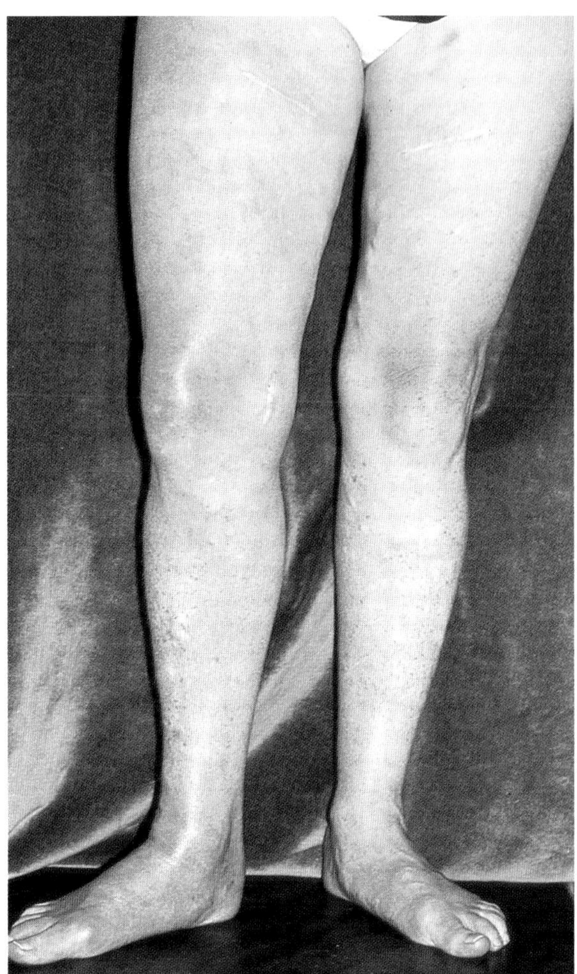

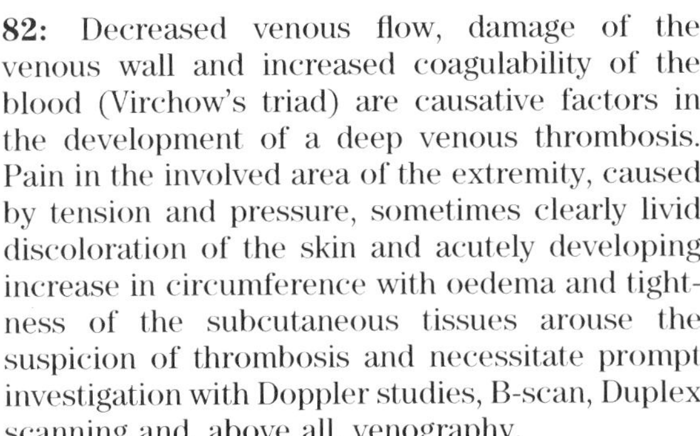

82: Decreased venous flow, damage of the venous wall and increased coagulability of the blood (Virchow's triad) are causative factors in the development of a deep venous thrombosis. Pain in the involved area of the extremity, caused by tension and pressure, sometimes clearly livid discoloration of the skin and acutely developing increase in circumference with oedema and tightness of the subcutaneous tissues arouse the suspicion of thrombosis and necessitate prompt investigation with Doppler studies, B-scan, Duplex scanning and, above all, venography.

83: With venous occlusion plethysmography, venous capacity and outflow can be measured in the upper leg from a change in circumference when occlusion is applied and suddenly released. The equipment is useful above all for the diagnosis and subsequent monitoring of venous thrombosis. Measurements in the arterial system can also be made.

84: Persistent difference in circumference and tendency to swell, in this case after pelvic venous thrombosis, indicate a venous hypertension as a result of valve destruction. Lifelong compression therapy is often necessary.

85: After treatment of the acute phase of a pelvic venous thrombosis, treatment with a proper stocking is absolutely necessary to prevent recurrent thrombosis and oedema.

86: The thrombotic occlusion of the deep venous system with resultant valve destruction often leads to a post-thrombotic syndrome years after recovering from the thrombosis. Secondary varices develop because of the insufficiency of the major deep veins. The CVI causes trophic skin damage, sometimes to the point of ulceration.

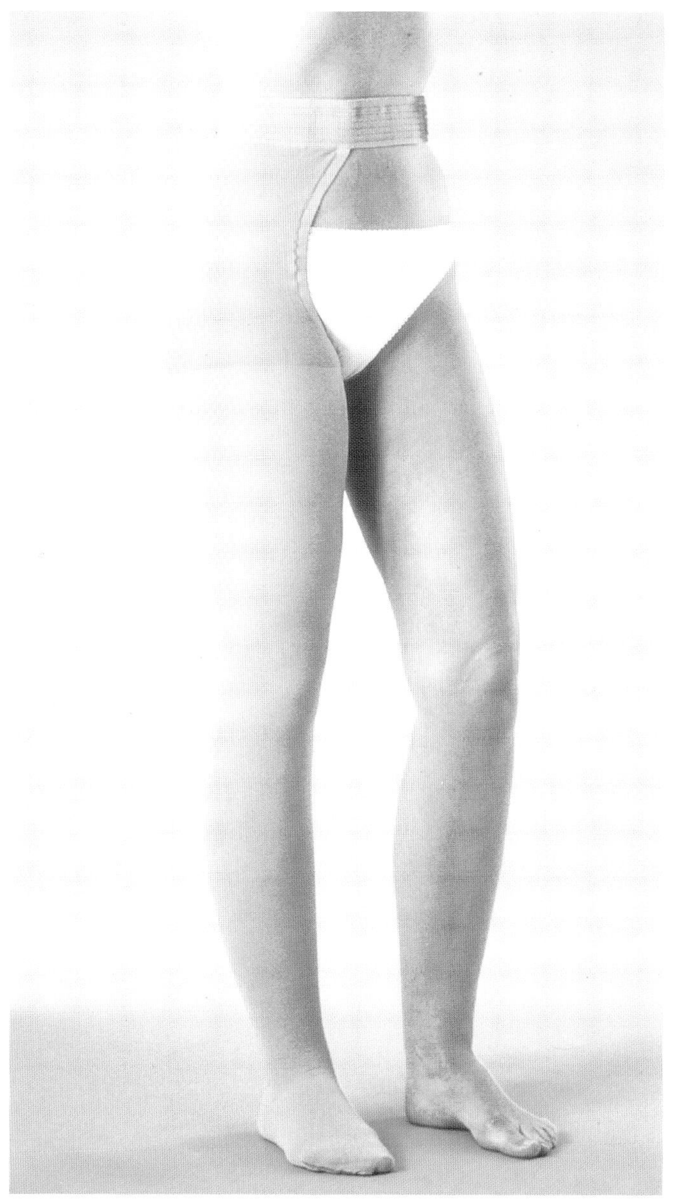
85

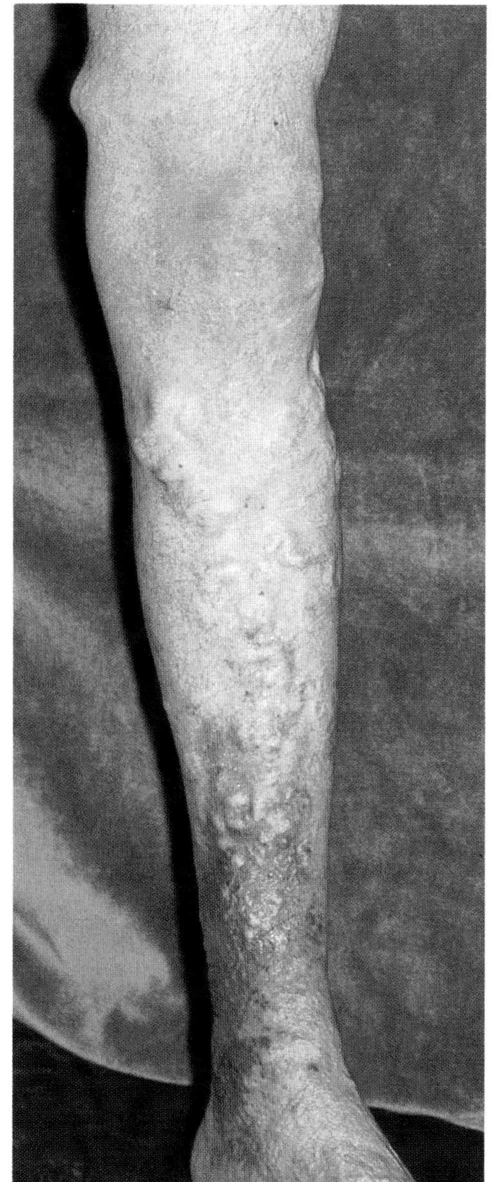
86

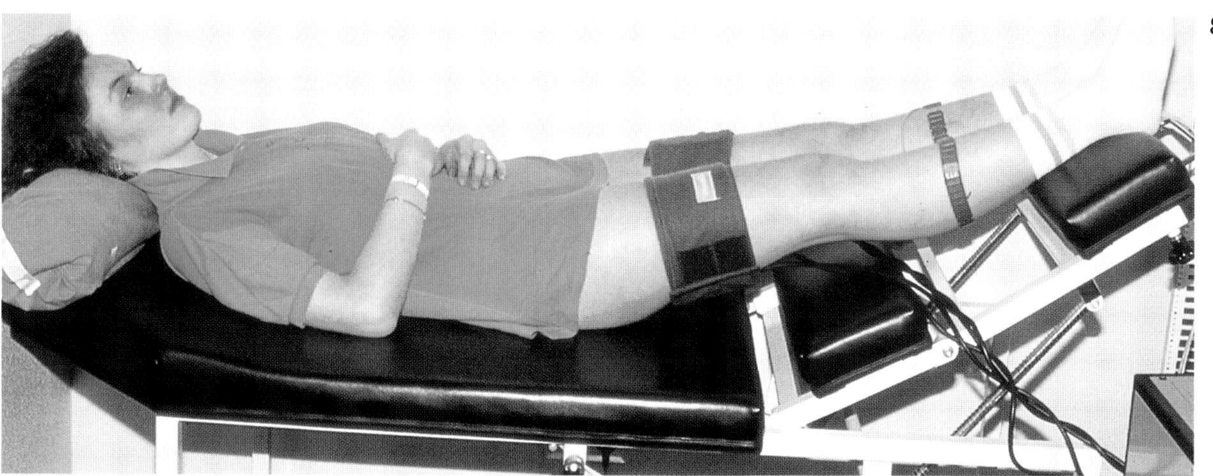
83

87

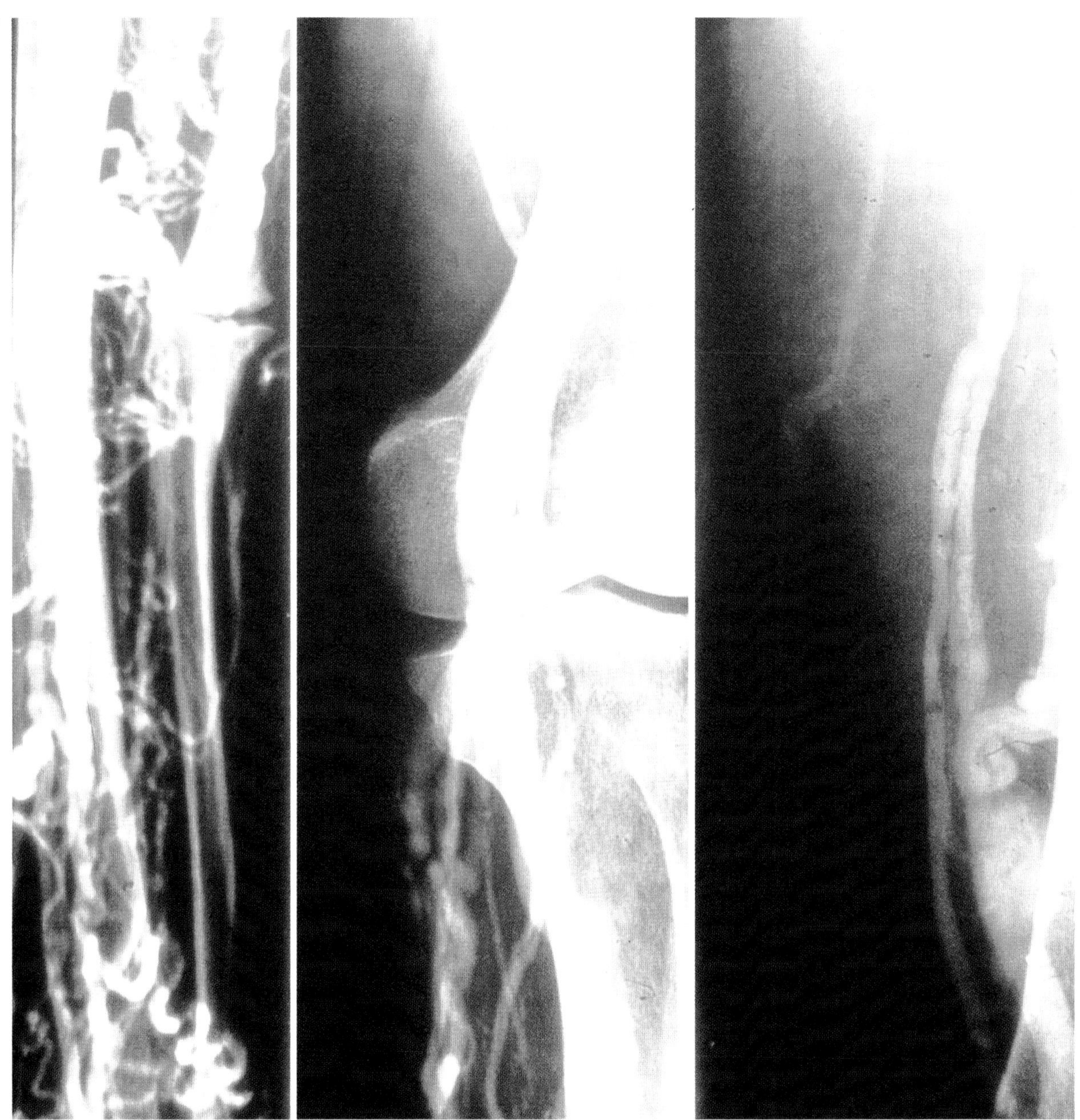

87: Good recanalization of the deep veins after thrombosis at the upper and lower leg level.

88

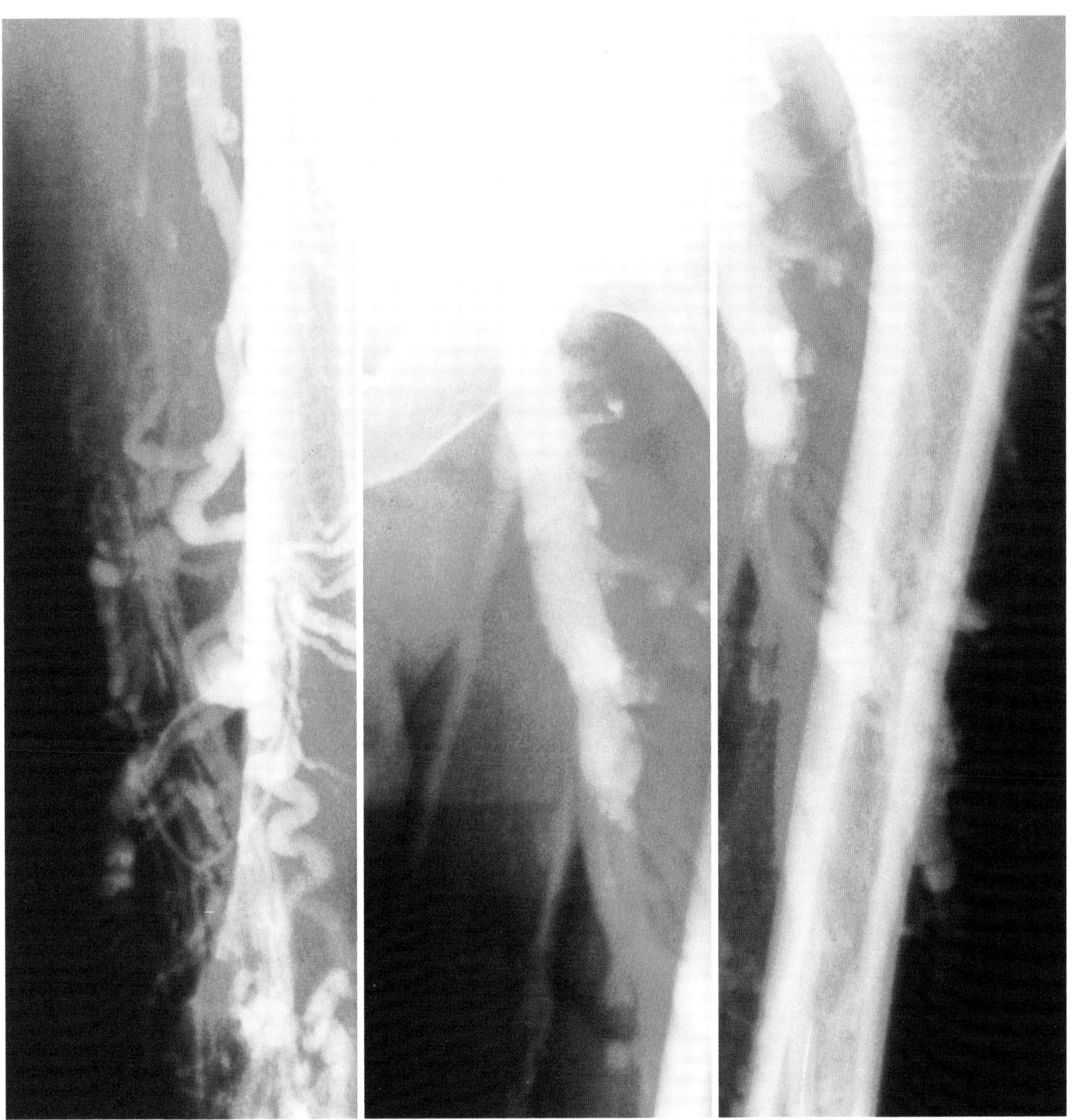

88: The radiological picture of a post-thrombotic syndrome is characterized by an irregular contour of the venous walls and obliteration of the lumen by areas of absence of contrast material as well as segments of scar-like narrowing or dilatation.

89

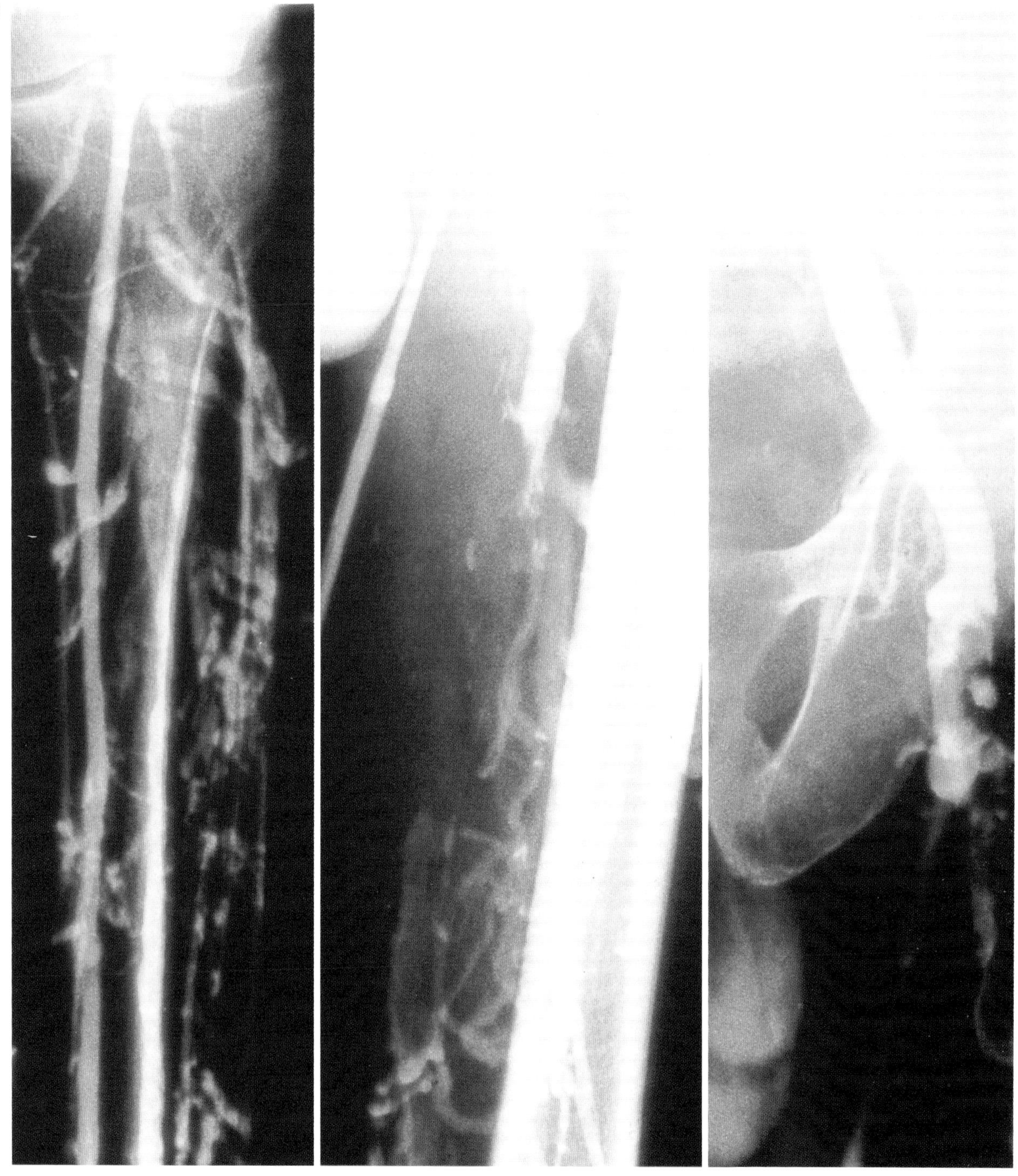

89: The picture shows a fresh deep vein thrombosis of the lower leg veins, the popliteal vein, and the superficial femoral vein up to the point of entrance of the profunda femoris vein, with collateralization into the long and short saphenous vein.

Venous ulceration

90: Cutaneous defects which are caused by inflammatory skin breakdown in the course of a varix are described as varicose, stasis or postphlebitic ulcers.

91: Varicose ulcers can be located over a cluster of varicosities in the ankle area. Ulcers are more often on the medial aspect of the lower extremity, but the lateral location is not rare.

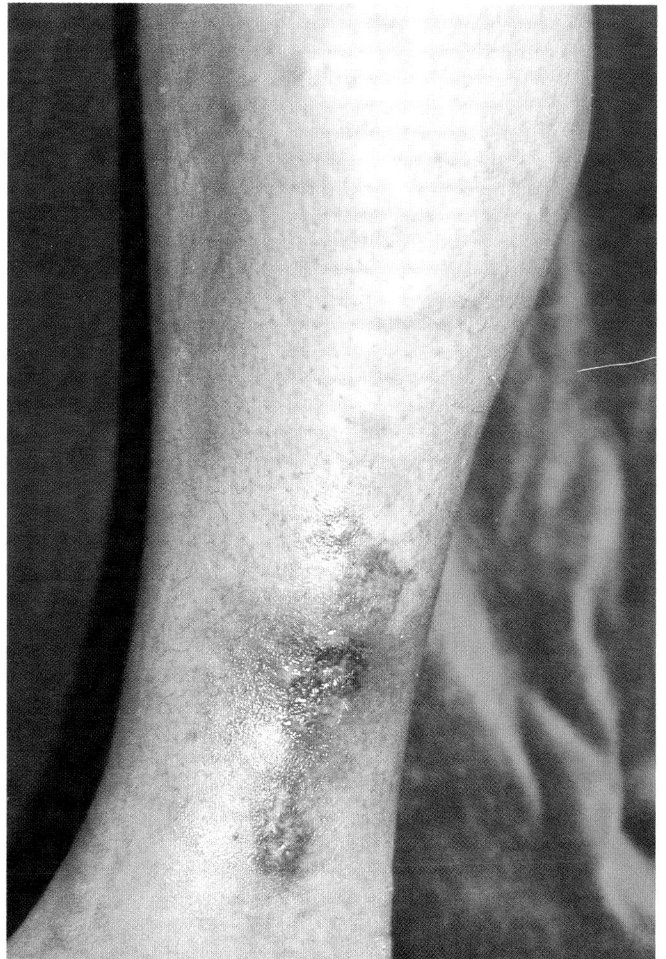

90

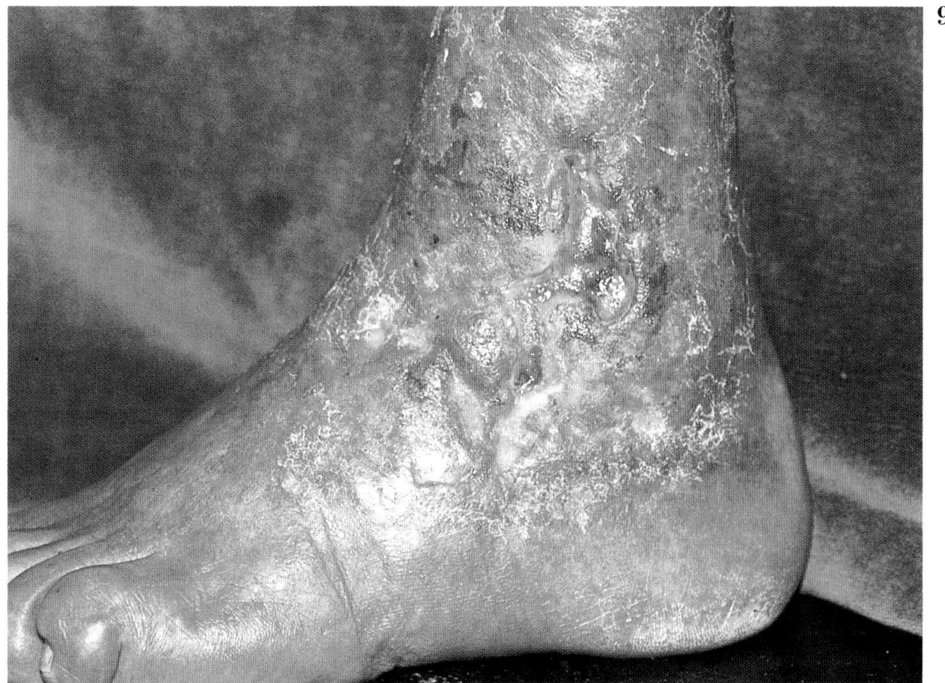

91

92

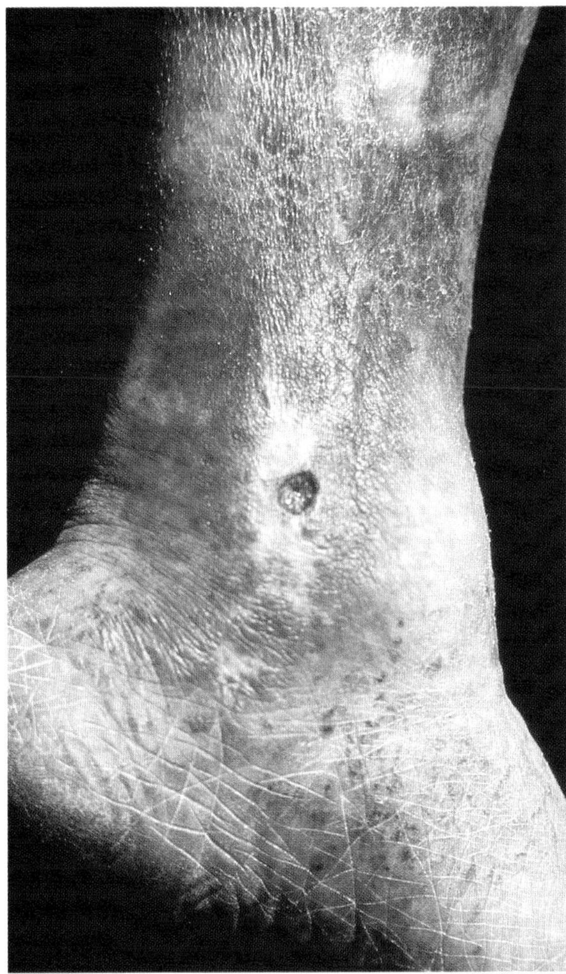

93

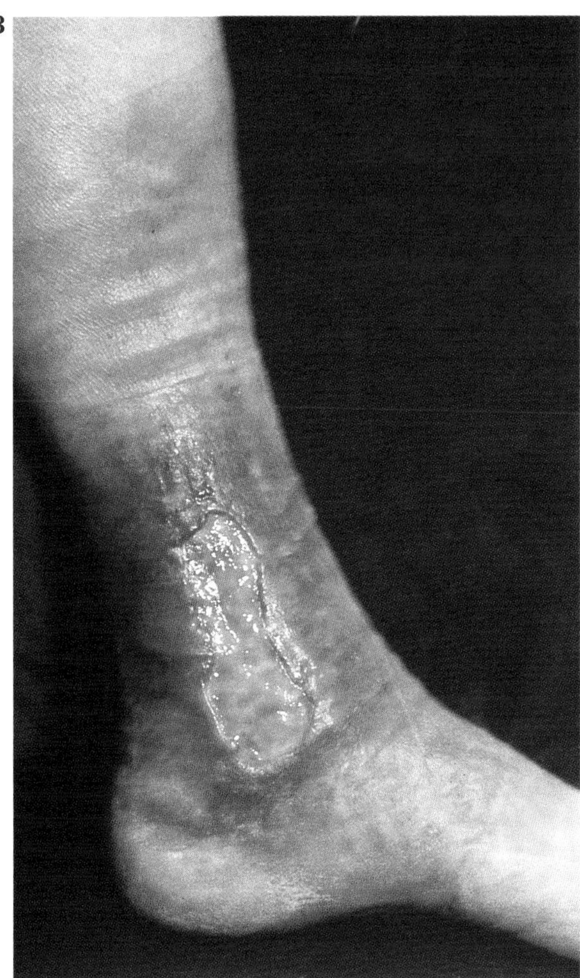

92: Ulcerations in an area of atrophie blanche are extremely painful because of co-existing local arterial hypoperfusion. If the pain is very severe, a short course of steroids can give some relief. The mainstay of therapy, however, is systematic compression. This can, in rare cases, reverse the hypopigmentation.

93: A blowout ulcer is caused by incompetence of the so-called Cockett veins with pre-existing trophic skin changes secondary to venous stasis.

94

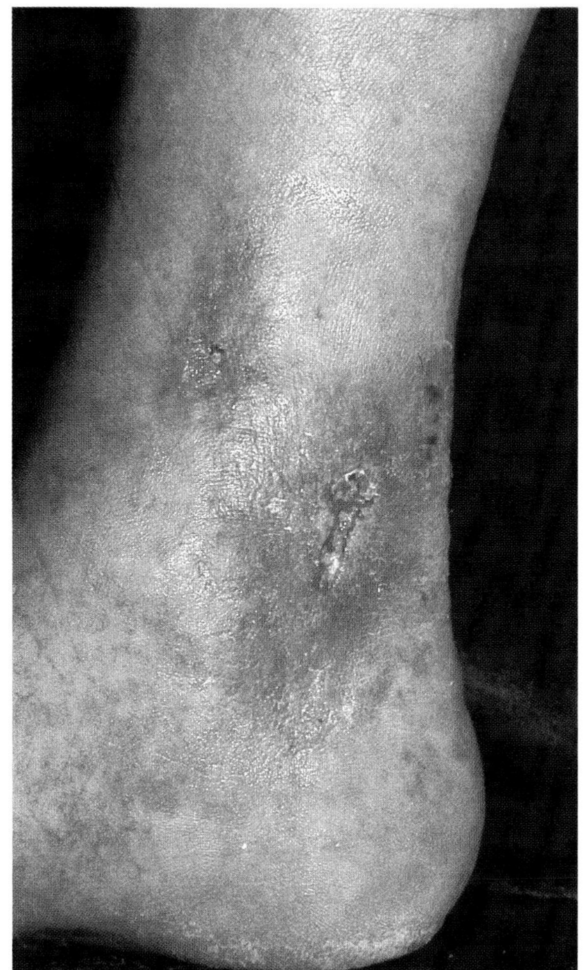

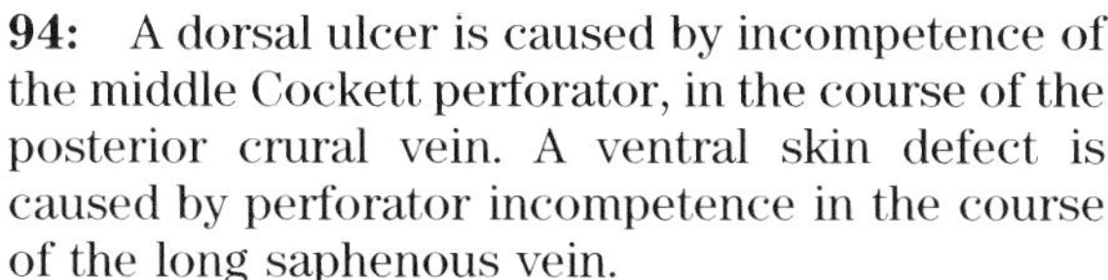

94: A dorsal ulcer is caused by incompetence of the middle Cockett perforator, in the course of the posterior crural vein. A ventral skin defect is caused by perforator incompetence in the course of the long saphenous vein.

95

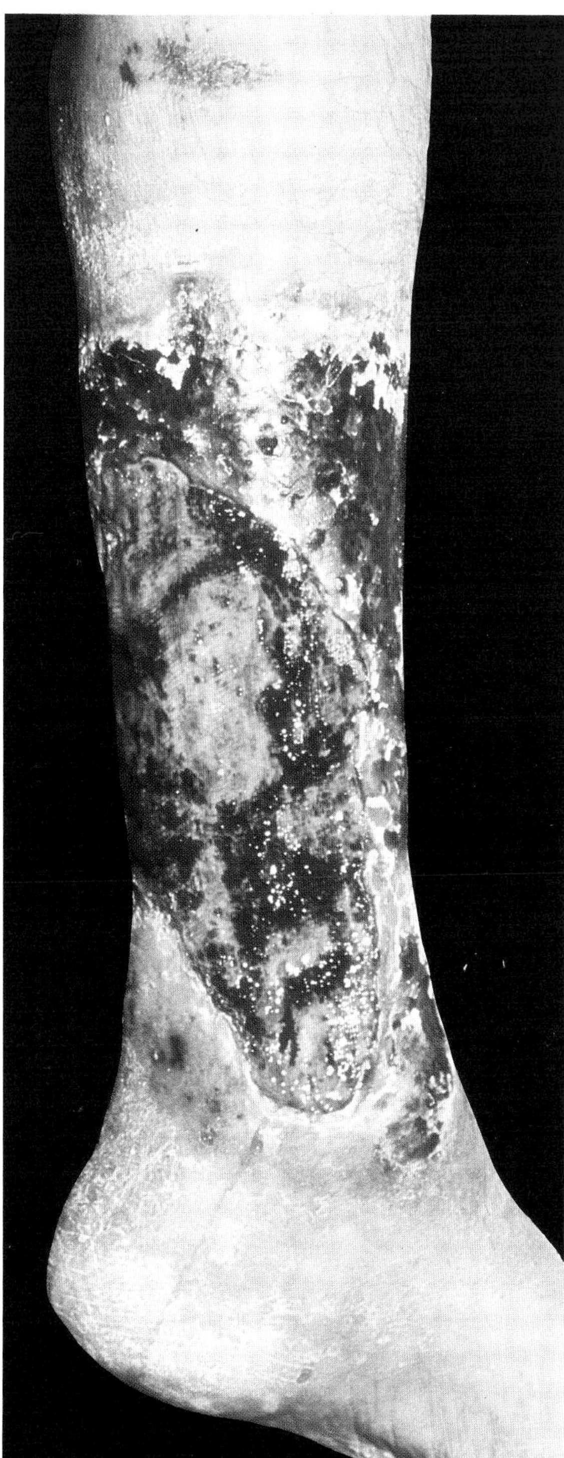

95: This extensive ulcer, encircling the lower leg, developed after a postpartum pelvic vein thrombosis and accompanying ankylosis of the ankle joint in a tiptoe position. It is an example of a joint-related venous stasis. The venous muscle pump cannot function because of joint damage.

96

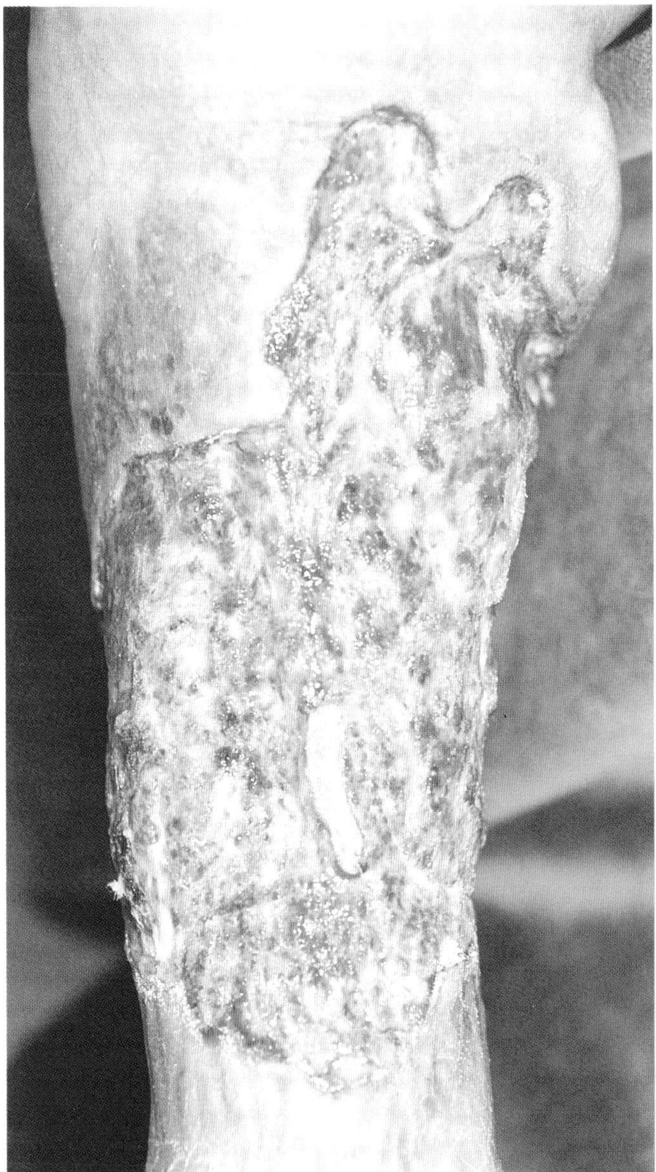

96: Extensive skin defects sometimes necessitate hospitalization with intensive local care and compression therapy, preferably supported by extensive physical therapy aimed at relieving the venous stasis. This includes intermittent compression, special exercises, compression bandages and manual lymphatic drainage.

97: Custom-cut foam rubber pads or ready-made compression pads exert pressure in the ulcer area and over the surrounding incompetent perforating veins. This leads to increased healing of the stasis ulcer.

97

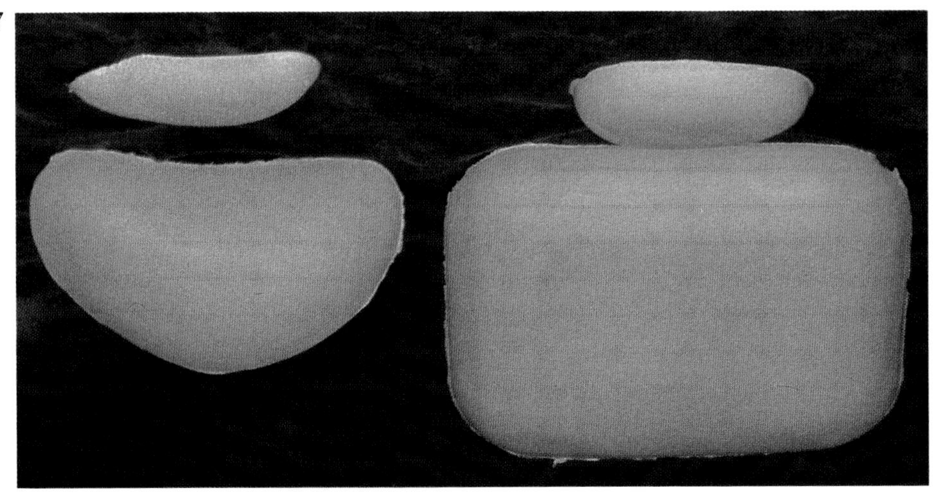

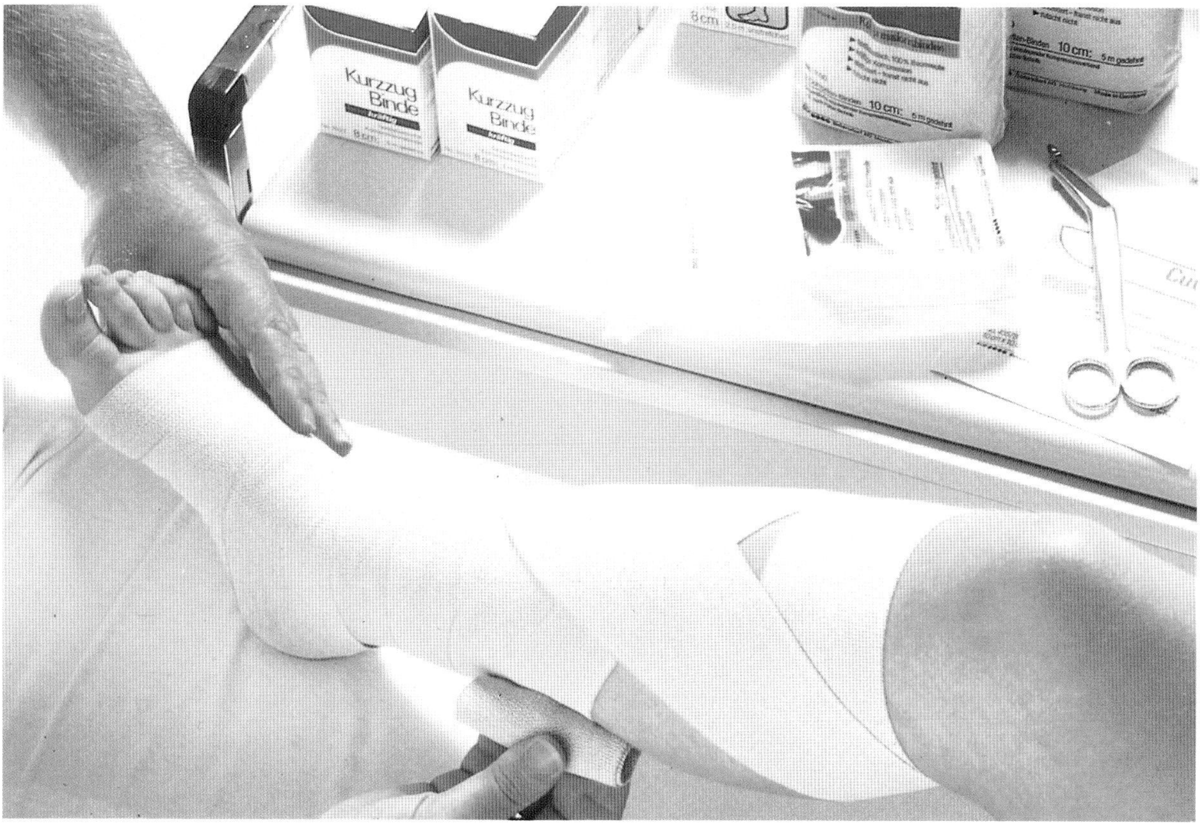

98

98: Compression therapy for stasis ulcer, venous oedema, and deep or superficial phlebitis as well as after sclerotherapy should primarily be accomplished by bandaging. Removable bandages should preferably have a high stretch resistance with low pressure at rest and high pressure at exercise.

99: Conspicuous skin defects of the lower leg or ulcers which do not heal in spite of intensive therapy should definitely be examined histologically. The histological diagnosis of the skin defect was lentigo maligna-melanoma Stage IV.

99

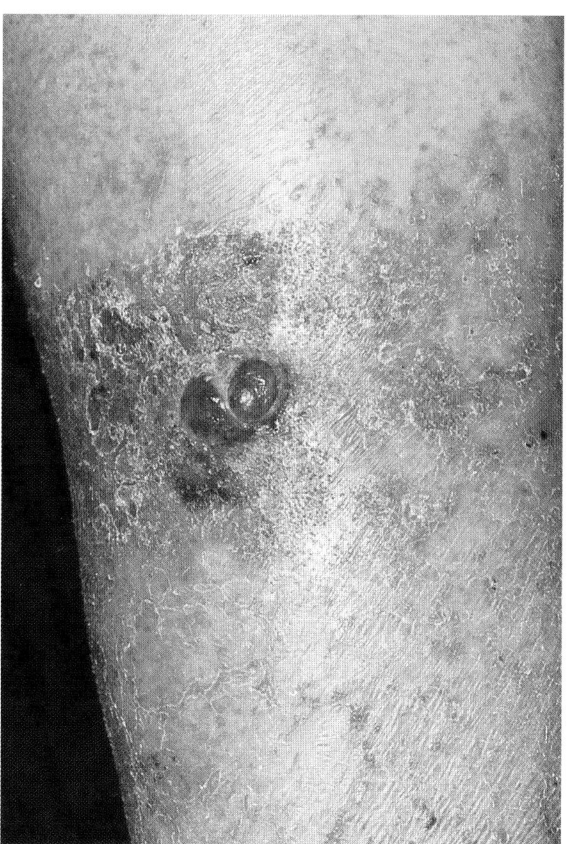

100

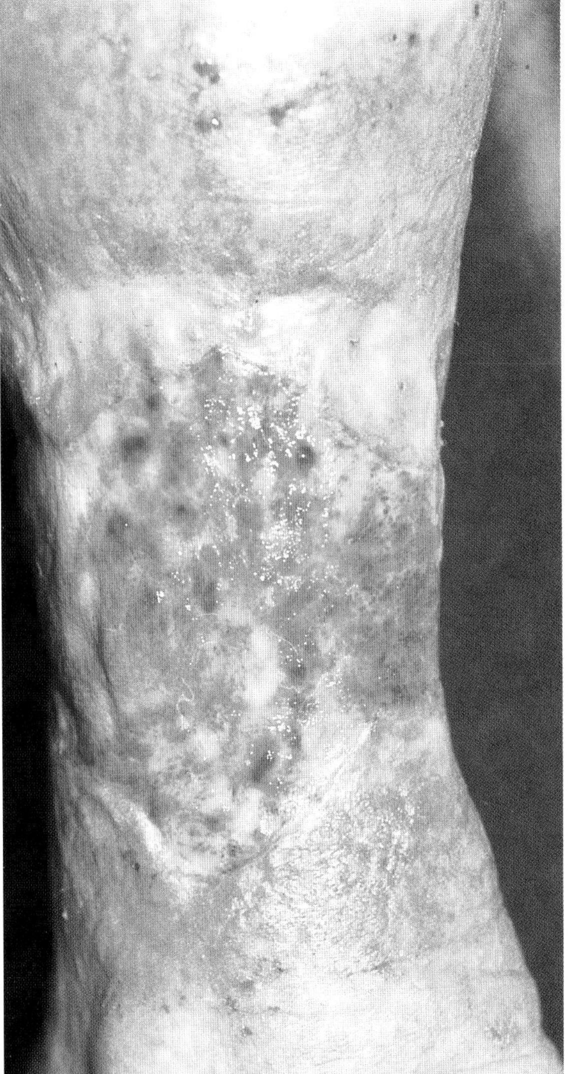

101

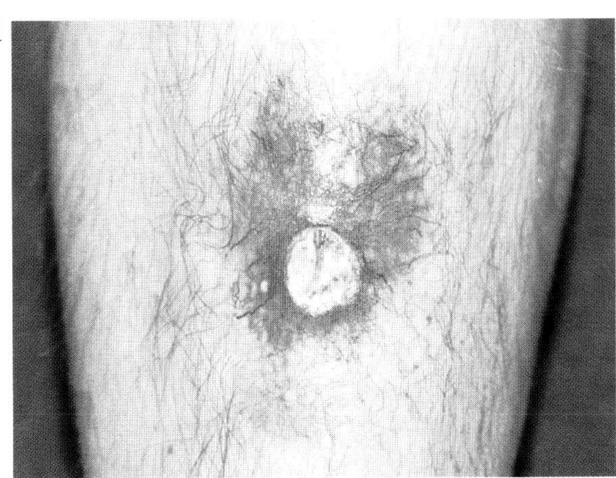

100: Although about 90% of lower leg ulcers have a venous aetiology, the differential diagnosis has definite therapeutic implications. Although the ulcer shown at first glance could be thought to be a venous gaiter ulcer, histological examination showed it to be a squamous cell carcinoma.

101: Necrobiosis lipoidica is characterized by brownish yellow foci, occasionally with central ulcerations. There is frequently a co-existing diabetes.

102: A mixed ulcer is caused by impairment of the arterial and venous flow. In addition to increase of the arterial inflow, for example through prostaglandin therapy, compression treatment with a pressure of 80 mm Hg or higher at the ankle, depending on what the patient can tolerate, can usually be given.

102

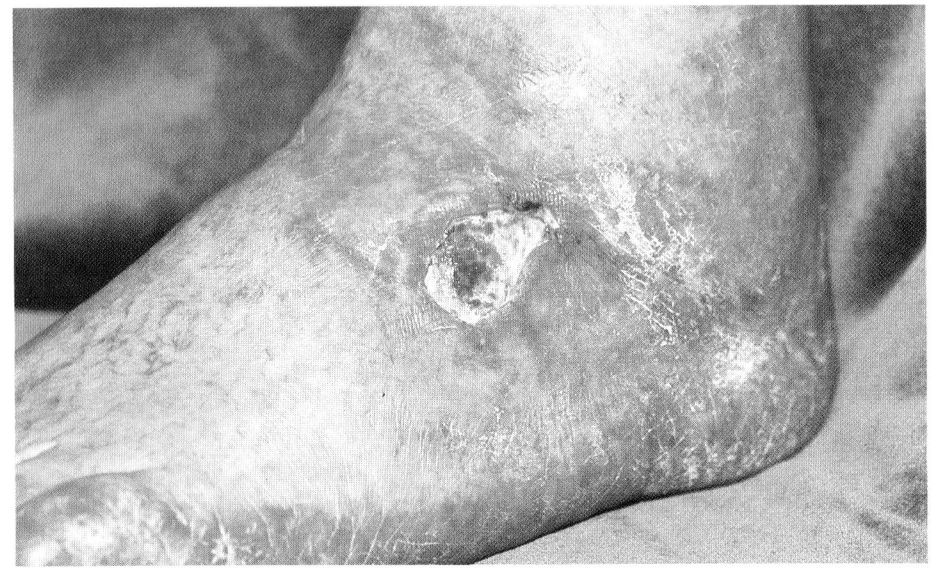

103

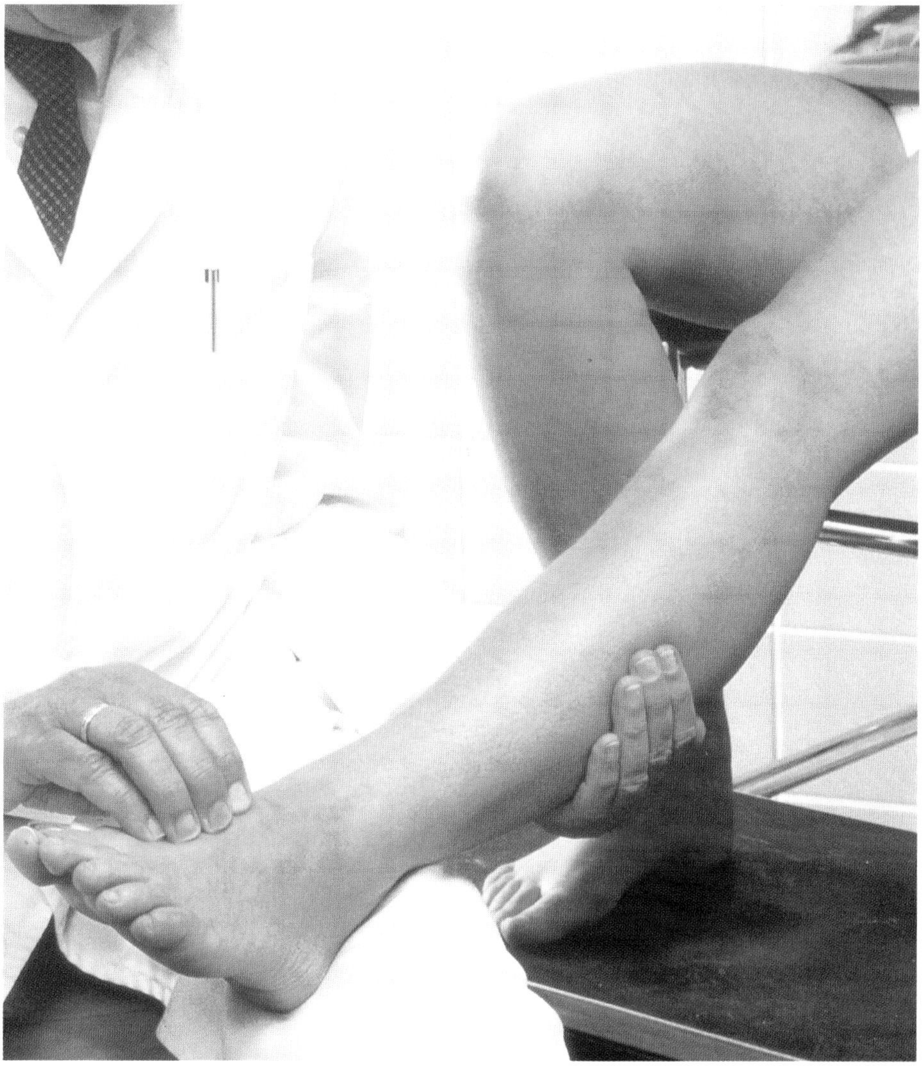

104

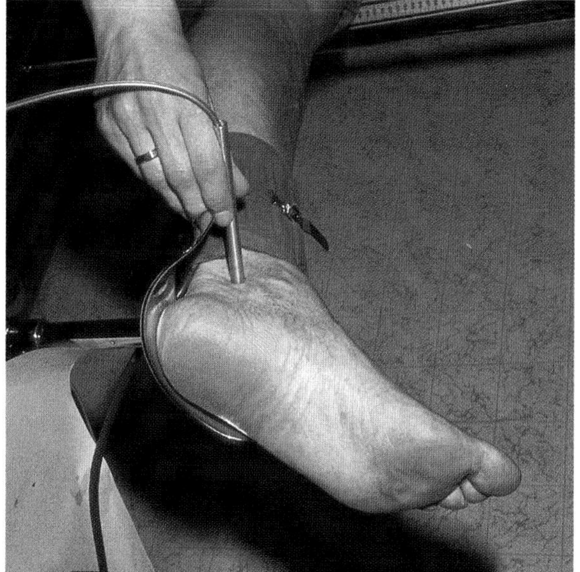

103: Palpation of the pedal pulses is part of every phlebological examination. This should include at least the dorsalis pedis artery and the posterior tibial artery.

104: When pedal pulses are absent or diminished or if the patient describes symptoms of claudication, one should immediately determine the pressure in the posterior tibial and dorsalis pedis arteries. The pressure should be as high as the systolic pressure in the brachial artery.

105

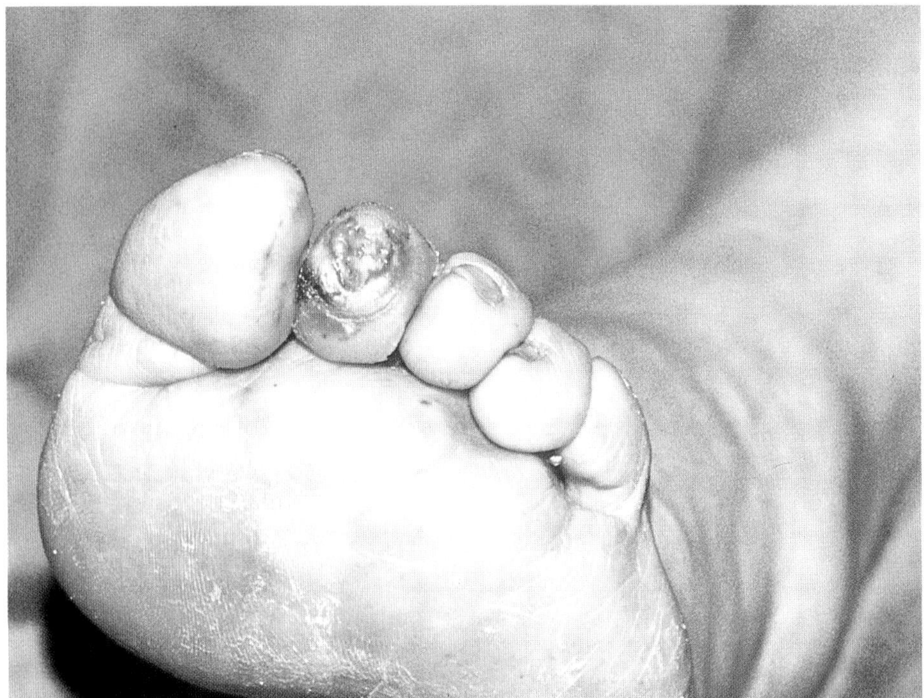

106

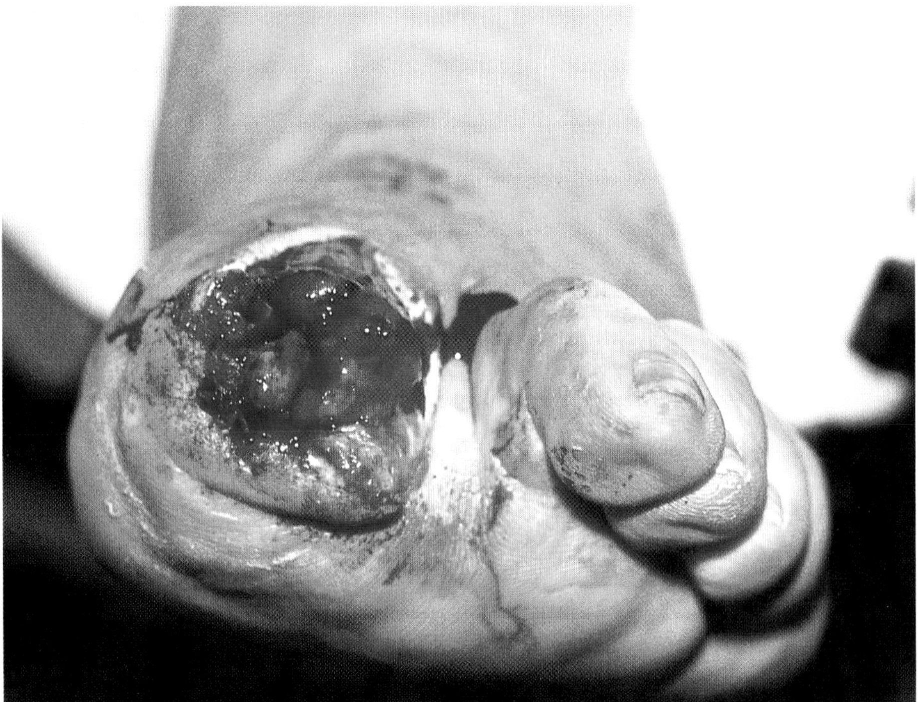

105: Diabetes mellitus, through macro- and microangiopathy, as well as neuropathy, leads to necrosis of the lower extremities, especially at the periphery. The lesions are sometimes completely painless.

106: Spontaneous amputation of the great toe at the metatarsophalangeal level due to diabetic gangrene. In addition to local care of the necrotic area, it is imperative to normalize the blood sugar level.

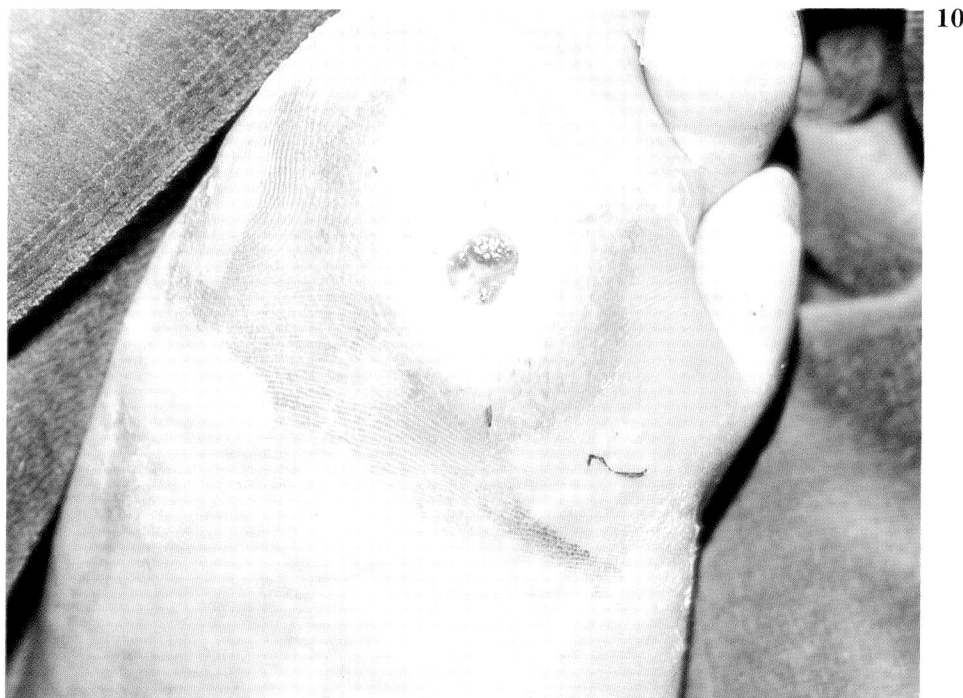

107

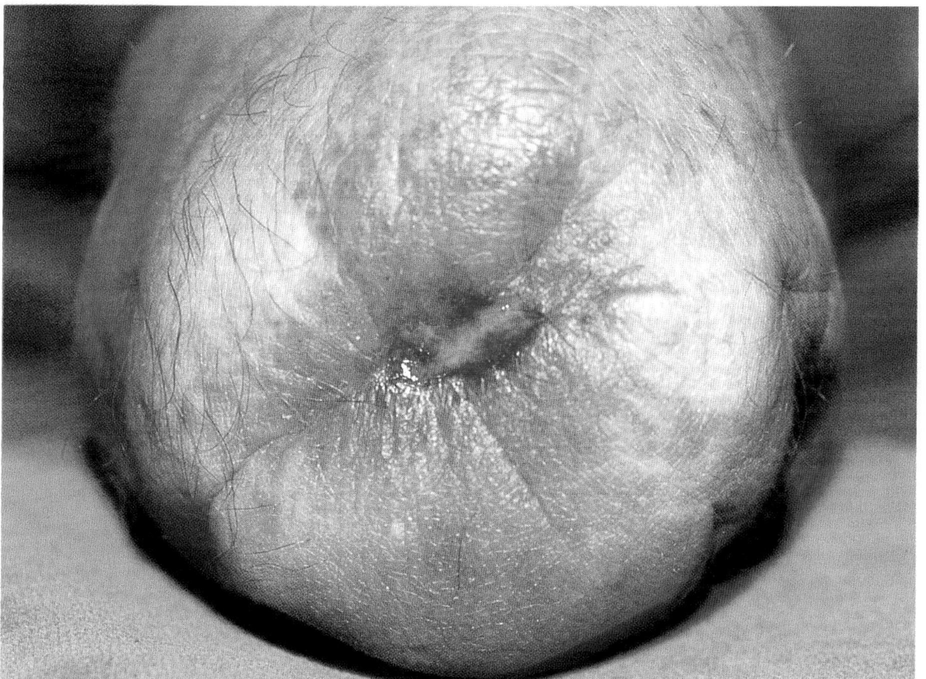

108

107: In skin areas with mechanical stress, microangiography and neuropathy in diabetes mellitus lead to a painless neurotrophic ulcer (malum perforans).

108: In this patient arterial occlusive disease Stage IV led to amputation of the lower leg. The pressure ulcer was caused by insufficient padding of the stump in the prosthesis.

109

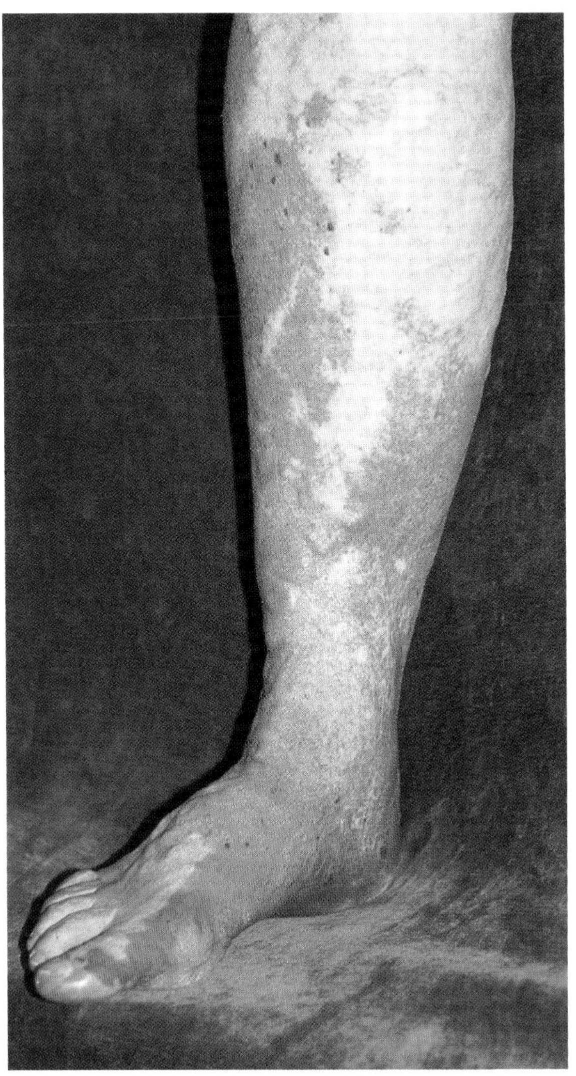

110

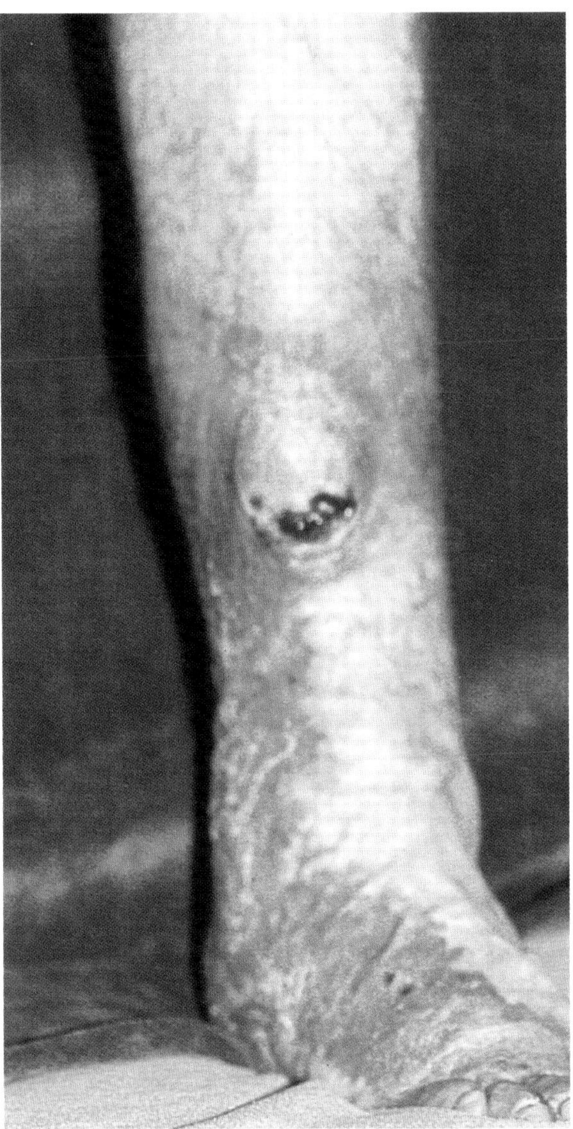

109: The Klippel-Trenaunay syndrome is a congenital angiodysplasia, characterized by the triad of (1) congenital angiectasias (nevus flammeus), (2) hypertrophy of the mesenchymal stroma with enlargement of an extremity, (3) varicosis caused by arteriovenous anastomoses.

110: In the Klippel-Trenaunay syndrome, lower leg ulcers can sometimes be found.

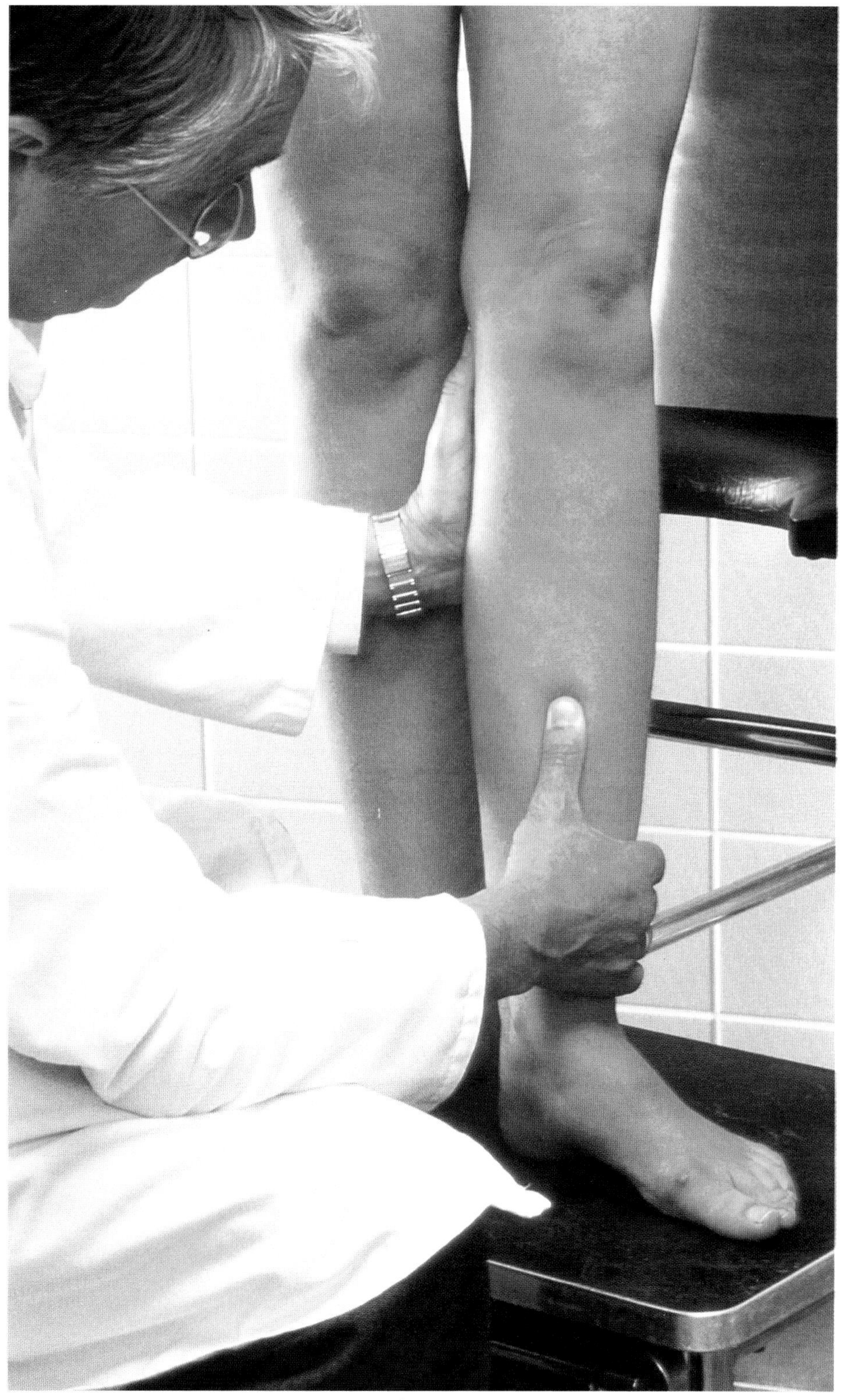

111: Every phlebological examination includes looking for oedema. The pitting caused by digital pressure should last for 30 seconds. Because of the often present periostitis of the lower leg, this examination can cause pain in a patient with venous disease.

112

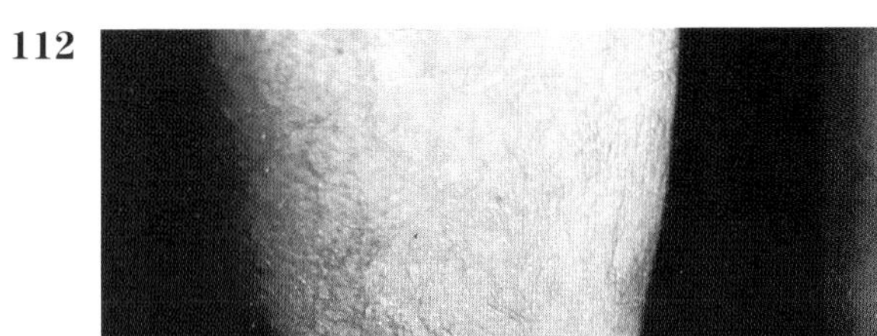

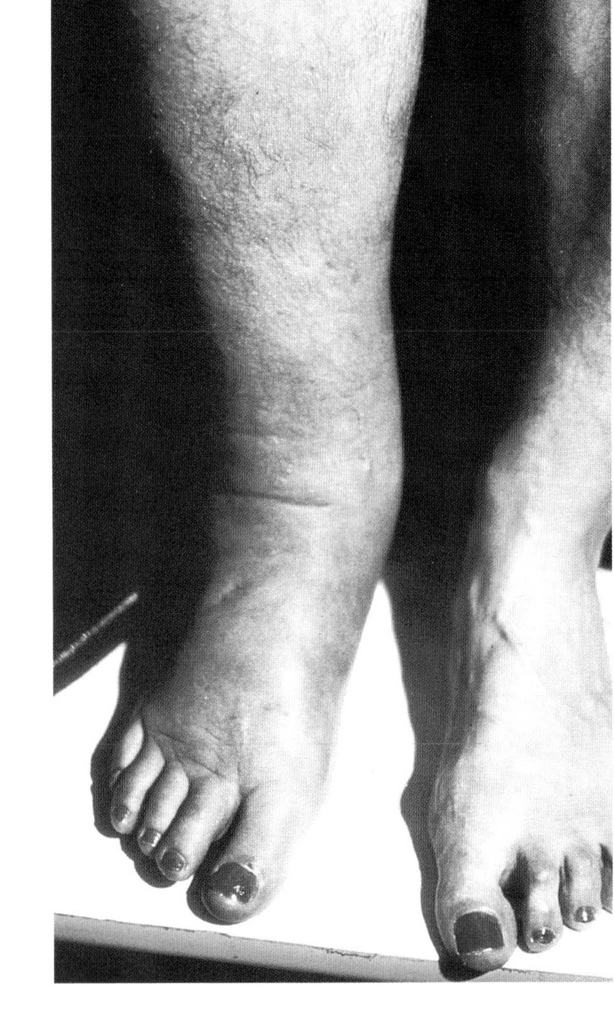

113

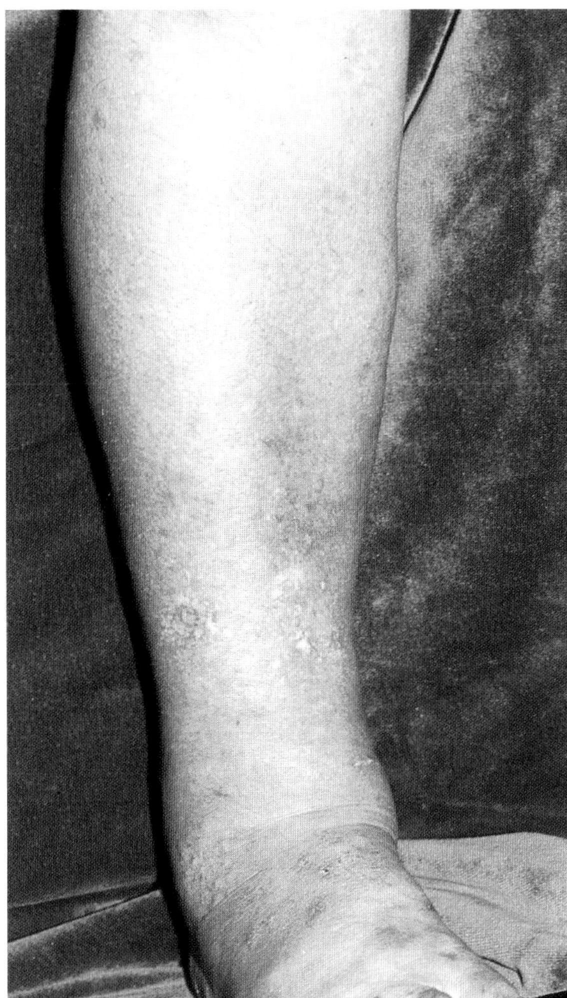

114

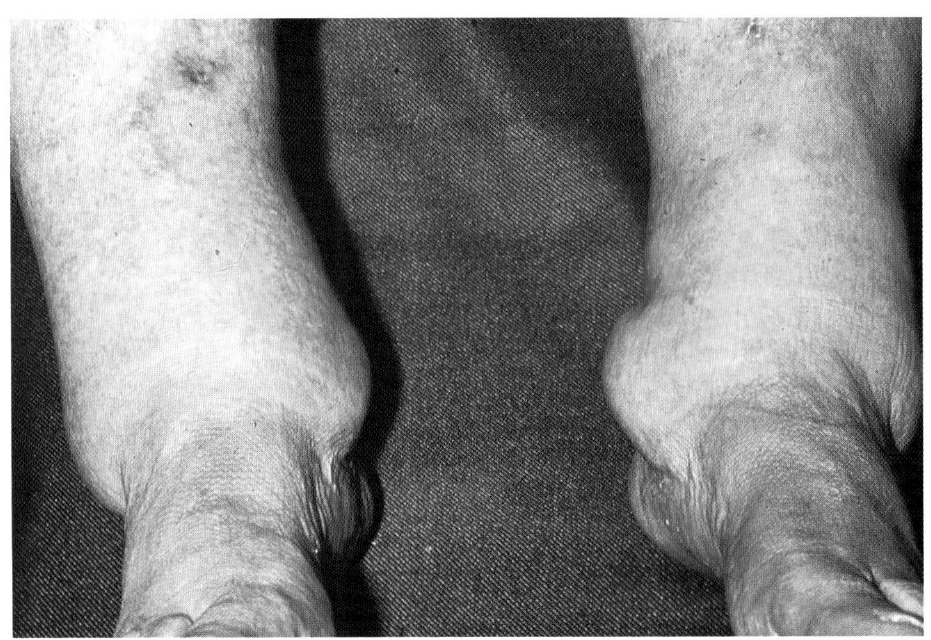

112: The aetiology of a unilateral oedema is usually venous, lymphatic, infectious or inflammatory after trauma. The history and clinical examination make the diagnosis easy. This case presents a venous oedema caused by acute deep vein thrombosis.

113: Chronic venous or lymphatic oedema can typically be seen in the spaces between the malleoli and the Achilles tendon.

114: In oedema of CVI, there are usually signs of trophic skin changes and there is also less involvement of the foot and toes. Cardiac and renal oedema, as well as bilateral oedema with other causes (e.g. protein deficiency or oedema caused by medication) are almost never accompanied by trophic skin changes.

115: Whenever an extremity has an increased circumference caused by venous disease, there is some lymphatic involvement because an oedema can only be formed if the lymphatic drainage capacity is overloaded. This can sometimes make the differential diagnosis between venous and lymphatic oedema difficult.

116: In lymphatic oedema, the distal foot and the toes are always also swollen. Stemmer's sign is positive, i.e. it is no longer possible to pick up skin folds from above the toes. In this case, the pits caused by digital pressure can still clearly be seen on the dorsum of the foot. If the condition continues, intravascular proteins are forced out into the interstitium and lead to fibrotic tissue changes, resulting in a persistent, rather doughy swelling.

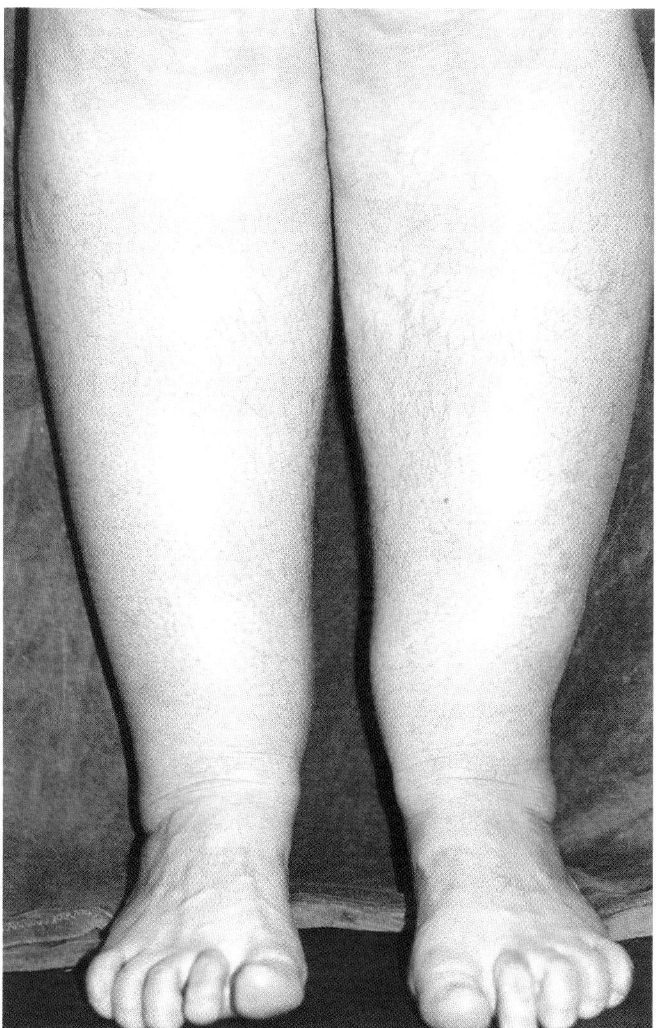

115

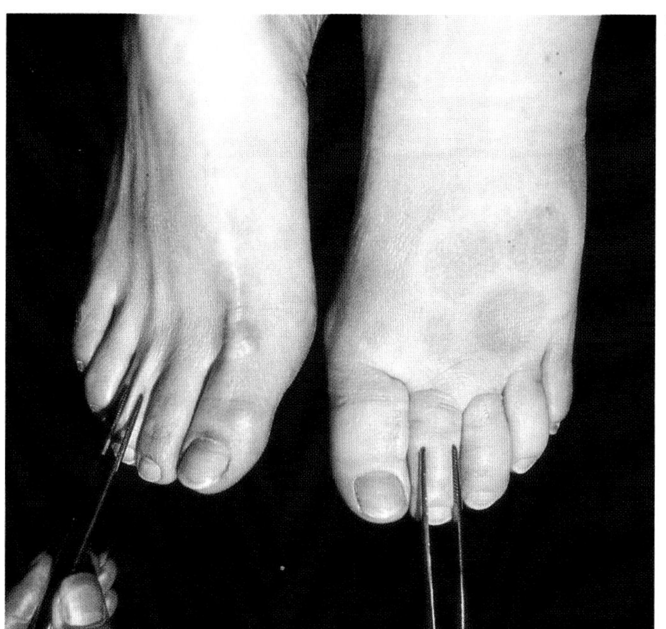

116

117

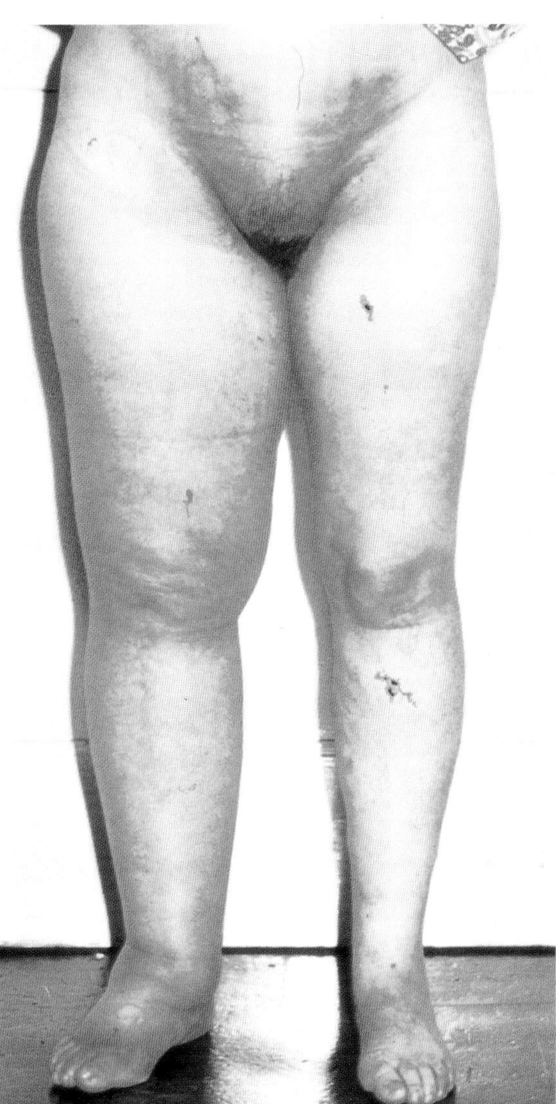

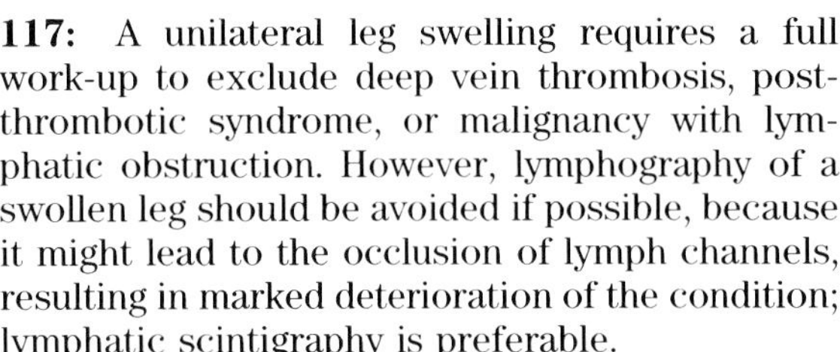

118

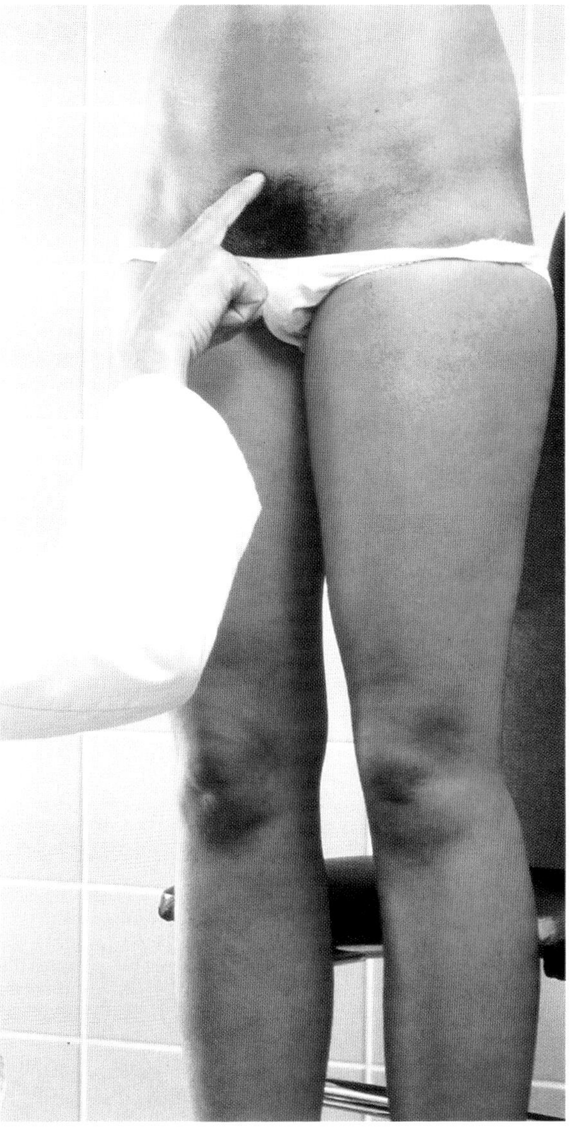

117: A unilateral leg swelling requires a full work-up to exclude deep vein thrombosis, post-thrombotic syndrome, or malignancy with lymphatic obstruction. However, lymphography of a swollen leg should be avoided if possible, because it might lead to the occlusion of lymph channels, resulting in marked deterioration of the condition; lymphatic scintigraphy is preferable.

118: It is necessary to palpate for enlarged lymph nodes as well as possible collateral veins, which suggest a unilateral pelvic vein occlusion.

119

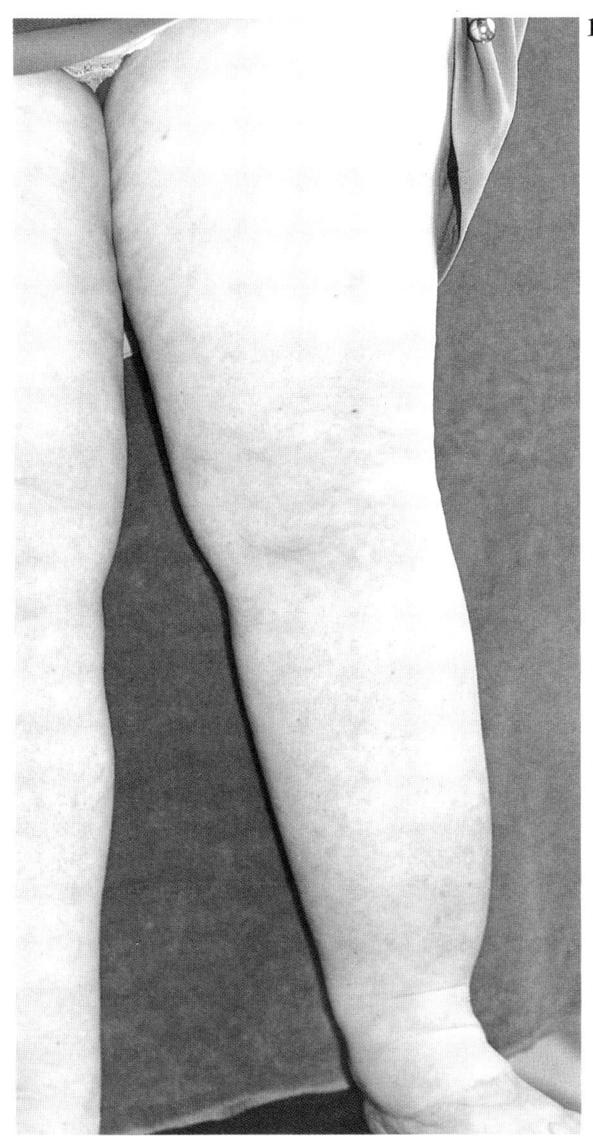

120

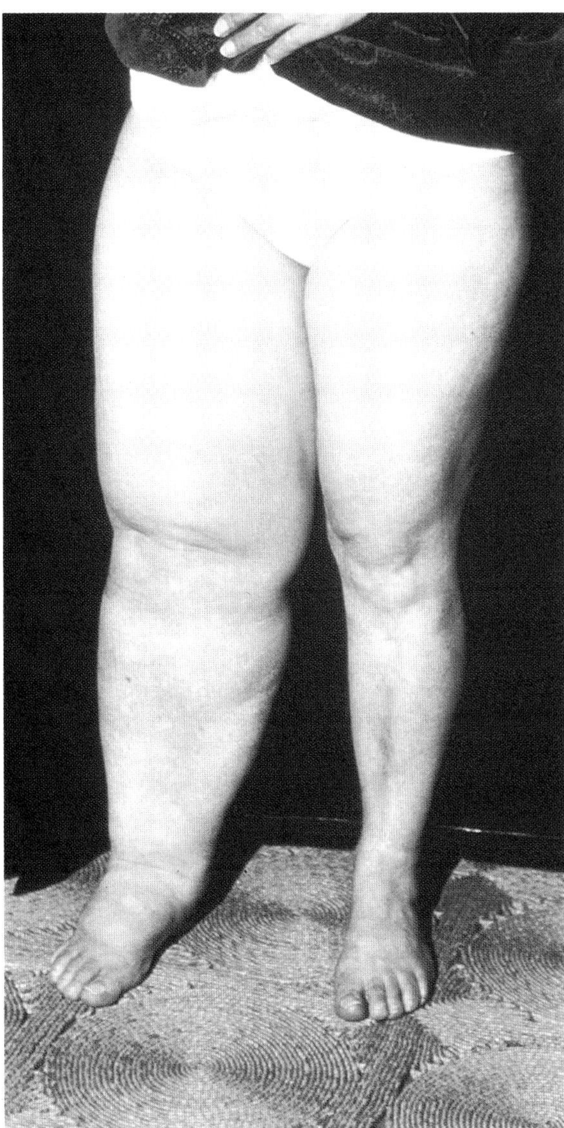

119: Until an underlying malignancy has been definitively excluded, mechanical compression methods to reduce the lymphoedema must be avoided because of possible embolization of tumour cells. However, compression therapy with bandages or stockings of compression Class IV is usually indicated.

120: Lymphoedema can be reduced with various forms of physical drainage therapy. Only when no reduction of circumference is accomplished in spite of intensive treatment, should a compression stocking of Class III or Class IV be custom-made, provided there are no contraindications such as impairment of the arterial supply.

121

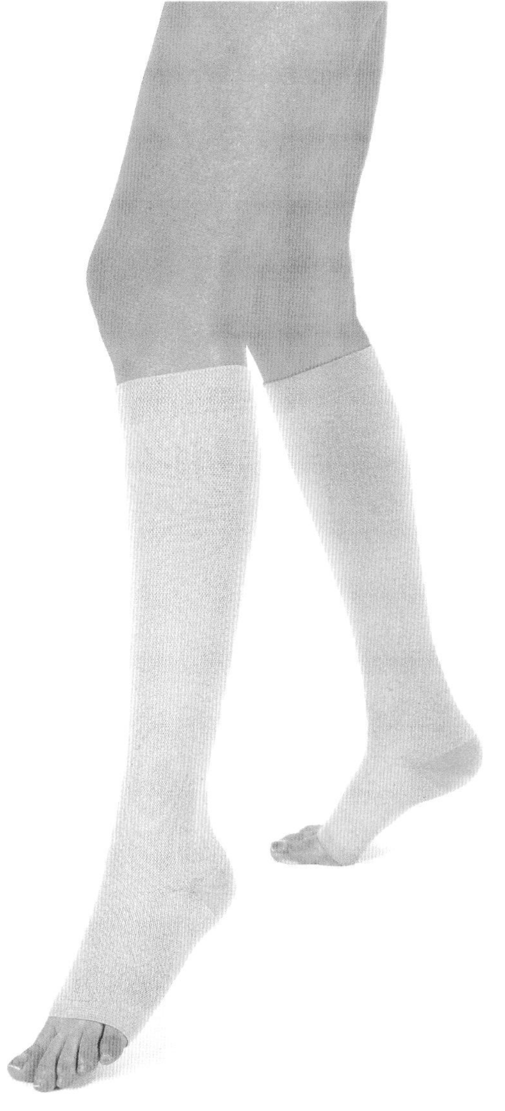

122

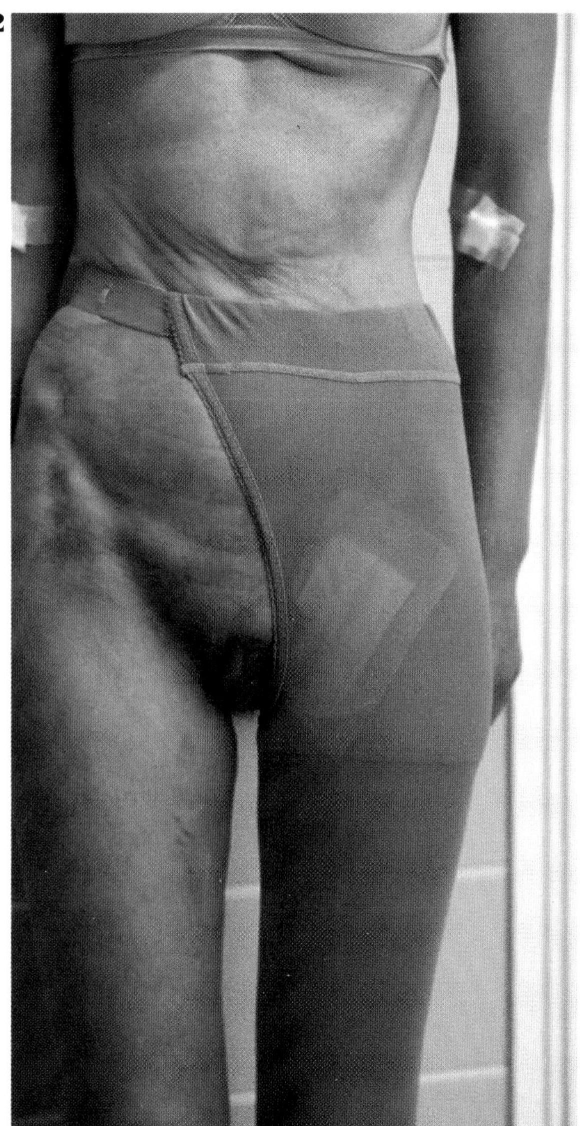

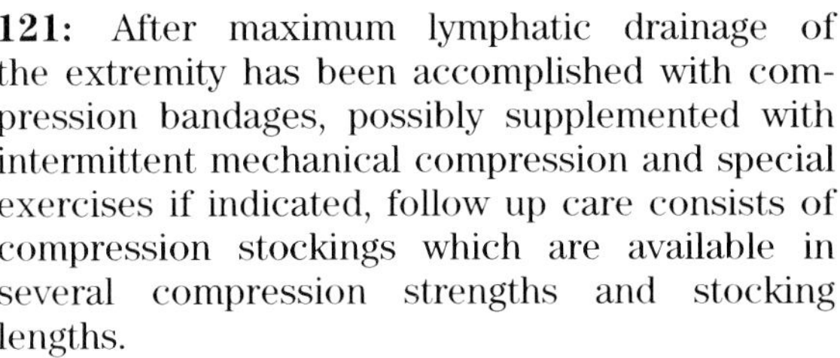

121: After maximum lymphatic drainage of the extremity has been accomplished with compression bandages, possibly supplemented with intermittent mechanical compression and special exercises if indicated, follow up care consists of compression stockings which are available in several compression strengths and stocking lengths.

122: After venous surgery such as, in this case, ligation and division of the long saphenous vein, a compression stocking with hip attachment, compression Class II, is prescribed.

123

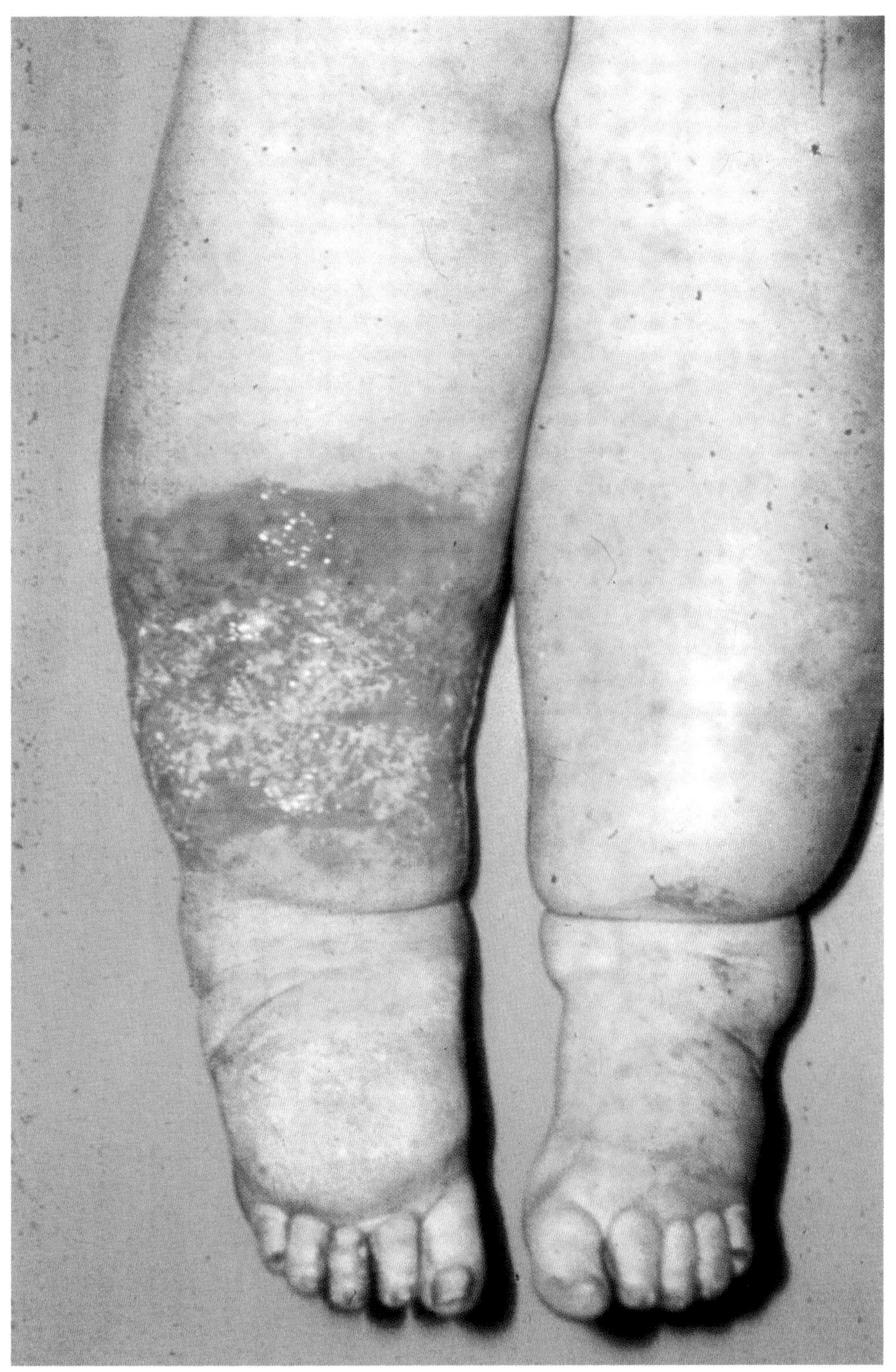

123: Erysipelas with an underlying lymphoedema should be treated with long-term antibiotic therapy.

124

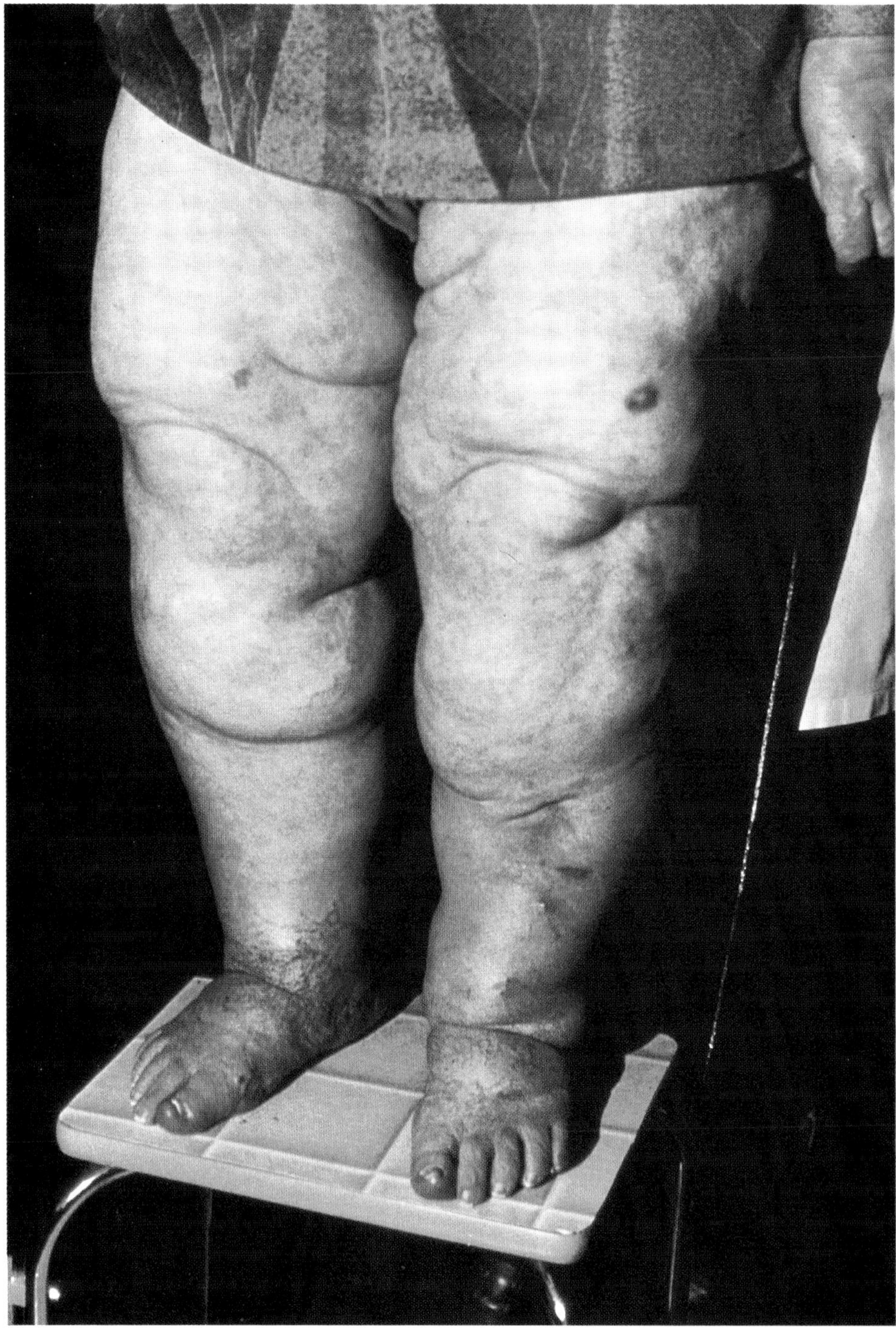

124: Lipoedema is most commonly seen in female adipose patients and it is usually bilateral. The firm swelling is most prominent in the proximal part of the extremities. Distally there is sometimes a fat collar above the malleoli, while the feet and toes are unremarkable.

3. Histopathology of the leg veins with special reference to phlebosclerosis

Reinhard Poche

The venous part of the circulation is divided into central or great veins (superior and inferior vena cava, pulmonary vein) and the peripheral veins, subdivided into intermediate and small veins. The veins of the leg belong to the so-called intermediate veins with a diameter between about 2 and 9 mm.

Differences in microscopic structure of vein walls depending on location and function

More than is the case with arteries, the morphological structure of veins differs from one area of the body to another depending on two circumstances: (1) the degree of hydrostatic pressure which the column of blood exerts on the wall of different veins, and (2) the mechanical requirements placed on the venous wall by the different surrounding tissues, such as loose or dense connective tissue, muscle or parenchymal organs (BARGMANN). In addition to this, the veins can also develop macroscopic and microscopic reactions to central circulation disturbances (congenital cardiac defects, primary and secondary right-sided cardiac failure, central arteriovenous shunts, etc.), and to peripheral circulation disturbances (ectasias or stenosis, stasis, thrombosis, peripheral arteriovenous fistulas, angiomas, etc.). These changes, consisting of hypertrophy of the musculature of the vessel and increase of elastic fibres, have been summarized in the term *morphological adaptation* (SCHOENMACKERS). The basic structure of any vessel wall, with intima, media and adventitia, is also found in veins. Nonetheless, it is not always possible to distinguish the borders between these three components as precisely as in arteries. There are, for instance, veins which have very little or no muscle component, so that a media for the most part is not developed at all (veins of the decidua, bone tissue, spleen, retina, brain, and cerebral membranes, skin, etc.). At the other end of the spectrum are veins which have a strongly developed muscular media and also smooth muscle fibres in the intima and the adventitia, where these are most often arranged in a spiral or longitudinal pattern, although these muscle fibres can sometimes also be found in a circular arrangement (iliac vein, femoral vein, popliteal vein, saphenous vein, cephalic vein, basilic vein, umbilical vein, median vein, internal jugular vein, some mesenteric veins, veins of the pregnant uterus, etc.) (BLOOM & FAWCETT, COPENHAVER). In the long saphenous vein this has caused some authors to consider some of those muscle fibres to be part of the media and, accordingly, some speak of an inner 'longitudinal media' and an outer 'circular media' (NEUMANN). Depending on their muscle and/or elastin content, one can differentiate between veins of the muscular type and veins of the elastic type (SCHOENMACKERS).

Age-related differences in the microscopic venous wall structure

Apart from the above differences related to location, function and adaptation, there are age-related differences in the histological structure of venous walls, which probably are only partially truly caused by age and partially genetically determined. Changes which are truly caused by aging consist generally of an atrophy of the smooth musculature and a corresponding increase in collagen connective tissue. Age-related fibrosis in veins often runs parallel with age-related fibrosis in arteries, but it definitely manifests itself clinically less often and it appears much later than the latter. It is sometimes impossible to make a clear distinction between so-called physiological age-related changes and pathological degenerative changes (ABRAMSON & TURMAN). The concept of 'physiological phlebosclerosis', used by many, seems therefore unnecessary.

Histological examination of the venous wall with analysis of the different structure elements such as endothelium, connective tissue cells, collagen fibrils, elastin fibers, myocytes, or smooth muscle fibres in the three basic structure components (intima, media and adventitia) in different age groups makes it possible to establish a histomorphologic aging profile of the different vein types (BUCCIANTE). It becomes evident that the well-protected deep veins, such as the femoral vein, show a relatively uniform aging profile, while in the mechanically much more stressed leg veins, e.g. the long saphenous vein, the aging profile is clearly more varied. However, the degree of structural modification in the peripheral small veins gradually diminishes distally. For the long saphenous vein the following aging profile has been developed (BUCCIANTE).

Collagen: In the *intima*, collagen fibrils appear after 15 years of age as subendothelial collagen pads which increase after age 60. In the *media* there are only a few collagen fibrils between the smooth muscle cells; these rarely increase in number, and only after age 60. In the *adventitia*, collagen fibrils are found from the outset; they increase more strongly after age 70.

Elastin: In the *intima*, elastic fibres appear already at age 8 and they can form an uninterrupted internal elastic membrane. (According to BARGMANN, only the large veins have an internal elastic membrane, while the small veins do not). At about age 10 additional subendothelial accessory membranes and individual elastic fibres are added, which later in life increase in number and thickness. In the *adventitia* the number and thickness of the elastic fibres increase visibly and constantly with increasing age.

Smooth Musculature: Longitudinal smooth muscle fibres, which are needed for strengthening of the venous wall, make their appearance in the *intima* by age 10 and increase until age 20. After age 70 there is often an involution of these smooth muscle cells. (According to embryologic studies by RICKENBACHER, these longitudinal muscle cells are laid down as early as in the third trimester of pregnancy). From the outset, the *media* consists of many circular smooth muscle cells which, starting at age 20, are mixed with collagen fibrils. In addition to this, longitudinal muscle cell bundles develop in the middle of the circular media from age 20 on, but later in life, usually after age 70, these can disappear again. In the *adventitia*, single spiral or longitudinal smooth muscle cell bundles are already present by age 8, but subsequently these increase only to a moderate degree. After age 50 there is a marked development of smooth muscle cells, which can turn the adventitia into the strongest part of the venous wall.
The appearance of longitudinal smooth muscle cells in the intima, media and adventitia and the hyperplasia of collagen and elastic fibres in the long saphenous vein are signs of adaptation, since these changes are less developed in the femoral vein and in the small peripheral veins. When evaluating the role of the microscopic structure of leg veins in disease, the pathological changes in the venous wall have to be considered in the context of these age-related variations in structure.

Pathology of the veins of the leg

Pathological changes take place on three levels, depending on the order of magnitude (POCHE): on the *macroscopic* level the pathological changes of the outer form (macro- or organ pathology) are examined with the naked eye or a magnifying glass; on the *microscopic* level the pathological changes of the tissue structure (histopathology, enzyme and immunohistochemistry, histophysics) are examined with light microscopy; on the *submicroscopic* level the pathological changes of the ultrastructure of the cells and organelles (submicroscopic pathology) are examined with the electron microscope.
In the **diseases of the leg veins** the main clinical interest is focused on those pathological changes which present themselves on the macroscopic level, and here varicose veins play the most important role. **Varicose veins** are discontinuous dilatations of veins, partly hose-shaped, partly spindle-or even barrel-shaped, saccular or knotty (to the point of forming an aneurysm), which can undergo lengthening and follow a tortuous course. Simple venous dilatations, which can be diffuse or circumscribed, are called venectasias.
Varicose veins are a very common condition. According to the 'Basle Study' (WIDMER et al.), a varicosis of the leg veins can be found in 55% of men and in 61% of women over 30, taking together all types and degrees of severity, although among these only 15% show a more or less clearly developed venous insufficiency. The varicosis can involve the main trunks of the leg veins, their tributaries and/or the small collecting veins down to the smallest vessels (spider veins).
Depending on their **aetiology**, we differentiate between primary and secondary varices. Of **primary varices** 77% are hereditary (LEU). Risk factors, which in the presence of an existing predisposition can cause a varicosis to manifest itself, include the following: congenital aplasias or dysplasias of the venous valves, a primary or secondary incompetence of the venous valves and/or other haemodynamic factors that lead to an increase of venous pressure, standing or sedentary occupation, age, obesity, chronic constipation, hormonal influences (e.g. contraceptives), multiple pregnancies, disturbances of the skin of the elasticity (e.g. striae), and toxic influences (e.g. alcoholism). **Secondary varices** develop through obstructions to the venous flow or disturbances in the distal outflow, which have to be bypassed by collaterals (e.g. thrombosis or thrombophlebitis).
In the **pathogenesis** of varices there is initially a venous congestion which can be local or can exist over a longer distance. This leads, via an increase of the venous pressure, and in the presence of the

postulated constitutional weakness of the venous wall, to discontinuous dilatations of the involved vein and thereby also to an ectasia of the commissures of the venous valves and as a result to relative valve insufficiency of the communicating and perforating veins (STAUBESAND). This leads to a further disturbance of the haemodynamics; the hydrostatic pressure on the venous walls increases, a stagnation of the venous outflow develops and finally a retrograde transfer of pressure take place, which leads to a reverse flow of the blood from the deep into the superficial veins, i.e. to an alternating flow between the deep and superficial system (WUPPERMANN & STROSCHE). The veins develop not only further dilatation and an increase in diameter of 1 cm and more, but also a lengthening and tortuosity, until a complete picture of severe varicosis has been reached.

Obviously these severe macroscopic changes have an effect on the **structure of the venous wall** and lead to pathological changes on the microscopic and submicroscopic level of the morphology. Because of the disturbed haemodynamics with chronic venous stasis, alternating flow of the blood etc., nutritional disturbances occur which have a profound influence on the cell metabolism and which are reflected in pathological changes of the ultrastructure of the cells and their organelles. In our subject, the microscopic level is of most interest, where the *histopathology of the varicosis*, resulting from the macroscopic, functional and submicroscopic changes, becomes manifest.

In the early stages of the varicosis, the intima of the venous wall is usually still delicate and thin and is in essence unchanged. In the media and adventitia, however, the disturbed haemodynamics and varying venous pressure very soon cause hypertrophy and hyperplasia juxtaposed to atrophy of the smooth muscle layer, which involves the circular as well as the longitudinal fibre bundles. The media and also the vein wall as a whole appear in some places thickened and in other places thin and irregular.

Initially there is no increase of connective tissue to be seen. There is still only a **varicosis without phlebosclerosis**. There are also no thromboses or inflammatory changes. The vasa vasorum are unchanged and can be followed down to the middle of the media. Occasionally small nerves or tactile bodies can be found in the adventitia, the importance of which is controversial (LEU).

In later stages there is also an increase of the collagen connective tissue, i.e. there is a **varicosis with phlebosclerosis**. The venous wall, similar to the arterial wall, reacts to a continuous unphysiological increase of intraluminal pressure with an increased synthesis of collagen fibres, first in the intima (*intimal fibrosis*), but then also in the media (*medial fibrosis*), and in the adventitia (*adventitial fibrosis*). The intima can thus show small flat patches, but also massive fibrous pads, a mild sickle-shaped, semicircular or circular connective tissue widening or a wide band-like **fibrosis of the inner layer** of the vessel. The medial fibrosis, which usually comes only very late, can show a reticular pattern that can be delicate, large, or even coarse. The adventitial fibrosis can consist of a slight increase of delicate collagen fibres or a marked widening caused by coarse collagen. In addition to this, parts of the venous wall can undergo fibrosis when smooth muscle fibres become increasingly atrophic and finally totally disappear (especially in markedly nodular and elongated parts of the vein), and are replaced by collagen fibres. But at the same time it is also possible that the increased venous pressure exerted on intact musculature acts as a stimulus for hypertrophy/hyperplasia in parts of the venous wall with less thickening; this can occur in the circular musculature of the media as well as in the longitudinal musculature of the intima and adventitia. The intima and adventitia can show a simultaneous increase in collagen as well as smooth muscle cells; this is described as a **fibromuscular phlebosclerosis**, and is termed **endophlebosclerosis** when the intima is mostly involved, and **periphlebosclerosis**, when the adventitia is mostly involved. Later the media can become increasingly fibrotic and thereby thinner, and this can range from a **diffuse reticular fibrosis** to a **fibrous atrophy of the media**. Fibromuscular endophlebosclerosis as well as endophlebosclerosis with local thickening and band-like circular fibrosis can cause narrowing of the lumen of the vein, while the fibrous atrophy of the media can cause weakening of the venous wall and thus lead to a further widening of the lumen. When all layers of the wall have become to a greater or lesser degree fibrotic and when the smooth muscle cells have progressively dwindled, the venous wall can withstand the increased hydrostatic pressure less and less, and an ever increasing nonelastic ectasia of the wall can develop, which can assume grotesque proportions and is then described as a **venous aneurysm**. In the areas of local fibrous thickening of the intima, delicate **elastic fibres** can develop in addition to the collagen fibrils. In agreement with BARGMANN, we were rarely able to demonstrate a continuous elastica interna (so typical for arteries), only equivalent structures. The media contains, in addition to the smooth muscle cells, a few elastic fibres, which in the presence of increasing fibrosis can disappear. In the adventitia, on the other hand, one finds usually numerous elastic fibres which increase in number and thickness as the varicosis and phlebosclerosis progresses, especially if there is at the same time a marked hyperplasia of longitudinal smooth muscle cells. When in later stages the fibrosis of the adventitia predominates, the elastic fibres, in the presence of increasing fibrosis, can also decrease and in the end disappear.

Even with advanced phlebosclerosis, the basic structure of the venous wall — with intima, media and adventitia — can usually still be recognized, as the terms endophlebosclerosis and periphlebosclerosis indicate. However, when this is no longer the case and the fibrosis has completely destroyed one or more of the three layers, the term **destructive phlebosclerosis** is used.

When a varicosis has existed for a long time, lesions of the endothelium can develop and agglutination of platelets can occur. These small **platelet thrombi** can be primarily organized by connective tissue and thus lead to increased fibrosis of the intima, as DUGUID has shown in the intima of arteries. The small platelet thrombi can, however, also become the starting point of **precipitation thromboses** which further decrease the vein lumen and in the end occlude it completely. In addition to this, the stasis in the congested veins can lead to a **coagulation thrombosis**, which can suddenly occlude the lumen. Precipitation thrombosis and coagulation thrombosis constitute complications of the varicosis, and usually cause a temporary clinical deterioration. Swelling, redness and pain can clinically imitate thrombophlebitis. In reality it is relatively rare for a varicosis to lead to a true **thrombophlebitis**, i.e. an inflammation of the venous wall with secondary thrombosis, whereby the infection is either haematogenous, caused by a septic pyemia, venipuncture or intravenous infusion, as part of a migrating thrombophlebitis (which is the systemic disease of the venous system), or is spread by continuity to the venous wall from the outside. Independently from this **acute phlebitis**, which usually attacks the whole venous wall, one can in a varicosis occasionally find single, widely dispersed, small, focal, chronically inflammatory round cell infiltrates, which should be described as a mild **chronic phlebitis with small foci**, but which have no true clinical pathological significance, and which above all do not lead to thromboses.

Most **thromboses** is a severe varicosis are noninfectious. However, they constitute an additional outflow obstruction and complicate the natural history of the varicosis. The centre of larger thrombi can soften into a sterile abscess which can lead to an early recanalization. The thrombi are **organized** from the vessel wall. Capillary outgrowths, macrophages and fibroblasts invade the thrombotic material, break it down and change it into granulation tissue capillaries, which also develop collagen fibrils and later turn into collagen scar tissue. This scar tissue always has small blood vessels and macrophages with haemosiderin, the iron-containing breakdown product of haemoglobin. Under certain circumstances some of the small blood vessels can become more dilated and can turn into small veins, which displace the rest of the organized tissue to a greater or lesser degree; this is described as organization with recanalization of the thrombosed vein. When during this process the remaining organized tissue has been reduced to a delicate weave of connective tissue which is inside the vessel wall, such vessels are called 'rope ladder' veins.

In cases of **destructive phlebosclerosis** the large fibrotic areas of the venous wall very often contain small blood vessels or small intracellular or extracellular deposits of haemosiderin, or both. This suggests that a destructive phlebosclerosis — if not always, then still in a majority of cases — is the result of a preceding thrombosis which is now completely organized into connective tissue, even when such a thrombosis is not mentioned in the patient's history and cannot be traced.

The large fibrotic, endophlebosclerotic pads of the intima, which can often be found at venous valves and in the area of arteriovenous fistulas, indicate that a locally active unphysiologically high intravascular pressure can cause marked local proliferation of connective tissue. An advanced endophlebosclerosis can also involve the **venous valves**. If this happens, the smooth musculature at the attachment of the valves can be replaced by fibrous connective tissue. The very fine and delicate stroma of the valve, which contains only a few layers of collagen fibrils, forms abundant collagen and develops a partial or total fibrosis and fibrosclerosis, i.e. a **venous valvular sclerosis**. The fibrosed valvular stroma can undergo hyaline degeneration and this can lead to a shrinking and shortening of the valvular cusps and thus also to valvular insufficiency. In the end, turbulence can develop under sclerotic valves, which no longer move back and forth in the bloodstream, and this can further facilitate the breaking off of thrombotic material. The thus developing subvalvular thromboses can become the starting point for larger thromboses. However, they can also become organized into connective tissue and thus increase the fibrous endophlebosclerosis.

Lipoid deposits and calcifications in the venous wall, especially in the intima, have been described in the literature, but they practically never occur in our very large phlebological histopathological research material. The same goes for inflammation of the vein. On the basis of these observations we agree with the opinion of THURNER and MAY, that **phlebosclerosis** is a disease which has no relationship to arteriosclerosis and that its **aetiology** is in essence a haemodynamic one. **Functional disturbances** such as venous stasis, local abnormal stress on the venous wall due to increased hydrostatic pressure, and local or generalized venous hypertension, lead to muscular hypertrophy of the wall and increase of collagen in all three layers of the wall. These conditions are very much present in a varicosis and for that reason one finds that phlebosclerosis is often present in a varicosis and is usually very advanced. **Thromboses**, which at the same time complicate the varicosis, can play an important role in the **progression** of phlebosclerosis. We should finally also mention **aging** as a contributing factor for the development of a phlebosclerosis. **Metabolic diseases**, such as hyperlipidaemia, hypercalcaemia, and **inflammations** play **no essential role** in the pathogenesis of phlebosclerosis.

Conclusion

When the macroscopic pathology and the histopathology of a varicosis is studied against the background of a haemodynamic disturbance, the varicosis is seen to be an affliction in which a functional change, i.e. a congestion with increase of the venous pressure in the lower leg veins, in the presence of a certain constitution, leads to the morphological change of a discontinuous phlebectasia, which in turn leads to valvular insufficiency of the communicating and perforating veins and to the formation of varices. This in turn brings about further functional disturbances such as the temporary reversal of the pressure gradient between the superficial and deep veins of the lower leg and the development of an alternating flow between the deep and superficial system. This results in nutritional disturbances of the venous walls themselves, but also of the soft tissues and especially the skin. At the same time, the increased venous pressure also causes micromorphological changes of the involved vein segments, which at first consist of a juxtaposition of hypertrophy/hyperplasia and atrophy. Later, a disproportionately marked collagen increase and also a quantitatively smaller increase of elastic fibres follow. Finally, a phlebosclerosis develops, manifesting itself in various forms, such as fibromuscular or fibrous endophlebosclerosis and periphlebosclerosis, diffuse reticular media fibrosis which can go as far as fibrous media atrophy, destructive phlebosclerosis and valvular sclerosis. At the same time, the varicosis can culminate in formation of an aneurysm. Complications such as platelet thrombosis, as well as precipitation and coagulation thrombosis lead to further functional deterioration and increase of the morphological changes. Thus a vicious circle develops, which is progressive and which in certain cases can only be broken by a well-directed operative intervention.

References

ABRAMSON, D. I., TURMAN, G. A.: Aging changes in blood vessels. In: BOURNE, G. H. (ed): Structural aspects of aging. London, Pitman Medical (1961).

BARGMANN, W.: Histologie und mikroskopische Anatomie des Menschen. Stuttgart, Thieme (1964).

BLOOM, W., FAWCETT, D. W.: A Textbook of Histology. 9th Ed. Philadelphia, Saunders (1968).

BUCCIANTE, L.: Microscopie optique de la paroi veineuse. In: COMEL, M., LASZT, L. (eds): Morphologie und Histologie der Gefäβwand. Basel, Karger (1966).

COPENHAVER, W. M.: Bailey's Textbook of Histology. Baltimore, Williams & Wilkins (1964).

DUGUID, J. B.: Thrombosis as a factor in the pathogenesis of coronary atherosclerosis. J. Pathol. Bact. **58**, 207 (1946).

LEU, H. J.: Histopathologie der peripheren Venenerkrankungen. Bern, Stuttgart, Wien, Huber (1971).

NEUMANN, R.: Histologie der Vena saphena magna unter dem Gesichtswinkel der Architektur-Pathologie. Virchows Arch. path. Anat. **229**, 479 (1937).

PLATZ, F.: Topographische und funktionelle Anatomie der arteriellen Hautversorgung am Unterschenkel: Eine präparative angiologische Studie. In: J. STAUBESAND, E. SCHÖPF (eds): Neuere Aspekte der Sklerosierungstherapie, Springer-Verlag, Heidelberg, (1990).

POCHE, R.: Die allgemeine Pathologie der myokardialen Herzinsuffizienz. In: ROSKAMM, H., REINDELL, H. (eds): Herzkrankheiten. 3. Aufl., S. 437. Heidelberg, Springer (1989).

RICKENBACHER, J.: Zur Entwicklung der Venen der unteren Extremität. Zbl. Phlebol. **5**, 6 (1966).

SCHOENMACKERS, J.: Pathomorphologie der Beinvenen und ihre hämodynamische Rückwirkung. Zbl. Phlebol. **4**, 166 (1965).

STAUBESAND, J.: Kleiner Atlas zur systematischen und topographischen Anatomie der Venae perforantes. In: COKKETT, F., KLUKEN, N. (eds): Die klinische Bedeutung der Venae perforantes. Ergebn. Angiol. Phlebol. **34**, 1. Stuttgart, Schattauer (1987).

THURNER, J., MAY, R.: Probleme der Phlebopathologie, mit besonderer Berücksichtigung der Phlebosklerose. Zbl. Phlebol. **3**, 404 (1967).

WIDMER, L. K., LEU, H. J., BREIL, H.: Zur Epidemiologie der Venenerkrankungen. Baseler Studie II. Zbl. Phlebol. **6**, 257 (1967).

WUPPERMANN, TH., STROSCHE, H.: Funktionsdiagnostik und Klinik der Venae perforantes. In: COCKETT, F., KLÜKEN, N. (eds): Die klinische Bedeutung der Venae perforantes. Ergebn. Angiol. Phlebol. **34**, 37. Stuttgart, Schattauer (1987).

125: Mild varicosis: varying thickness of the muscularis of the media with mild irregularity of the lumen. Cushions of longitudinal smooth muscle cells in the intima. No true increase of collagen in the intima and media. Mild but definite increase of the longitudinal smooth muscle fibres, collagen fibrils and elastic fibres in the adventitia (fibrous-elastic-muscular periphlebosclerosis).
Segment of the left long saphenous vein of a 55-year-old woman (the patient also had a marked varicosis with phlebosclerosis, aneurysmal dilatation and thrombosis of the left Dodd perforator, which however is not shown here), (E.-#4204/90 I). ElHvG (Elastica-Hematoxylin-van Gieson). Magnif. 1.25 × objective.

126: Moderate to marked varicosis with mild phlebosclerosis: a mixture of hypertrophy/hyperplasia and atrophy in the muscularis of the media; the lumen shows moderate dilatation and local outpouchings. Flat fibrous cushions of the intima (mild fibrous endophlebosclerosis). Mild increase of collagen in the muscularis of the media. Combination of loose adventitia at the level of the thinned parts of the wall and stronger fibrous-elastic-muscular thickening of the adventitia (circumscribed periphlebosclerosis) at the level of the thickened parts of the media.
Segment of the right long saphenous vein with tributary of a 41-year-old woman (in this patient the varicosis was bilateral, both sides were operated on). (E.-#3616/90 I). ElHvG. Magnif. 1.25 × objective.

125

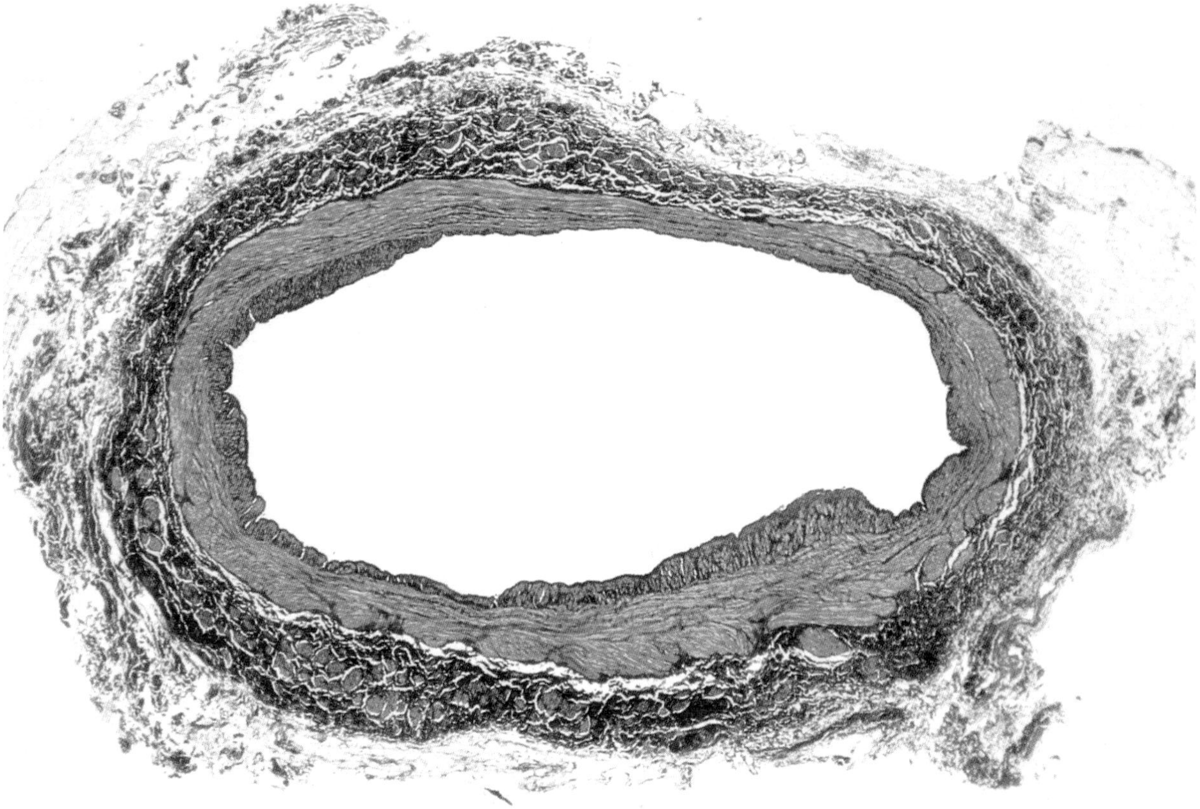

126

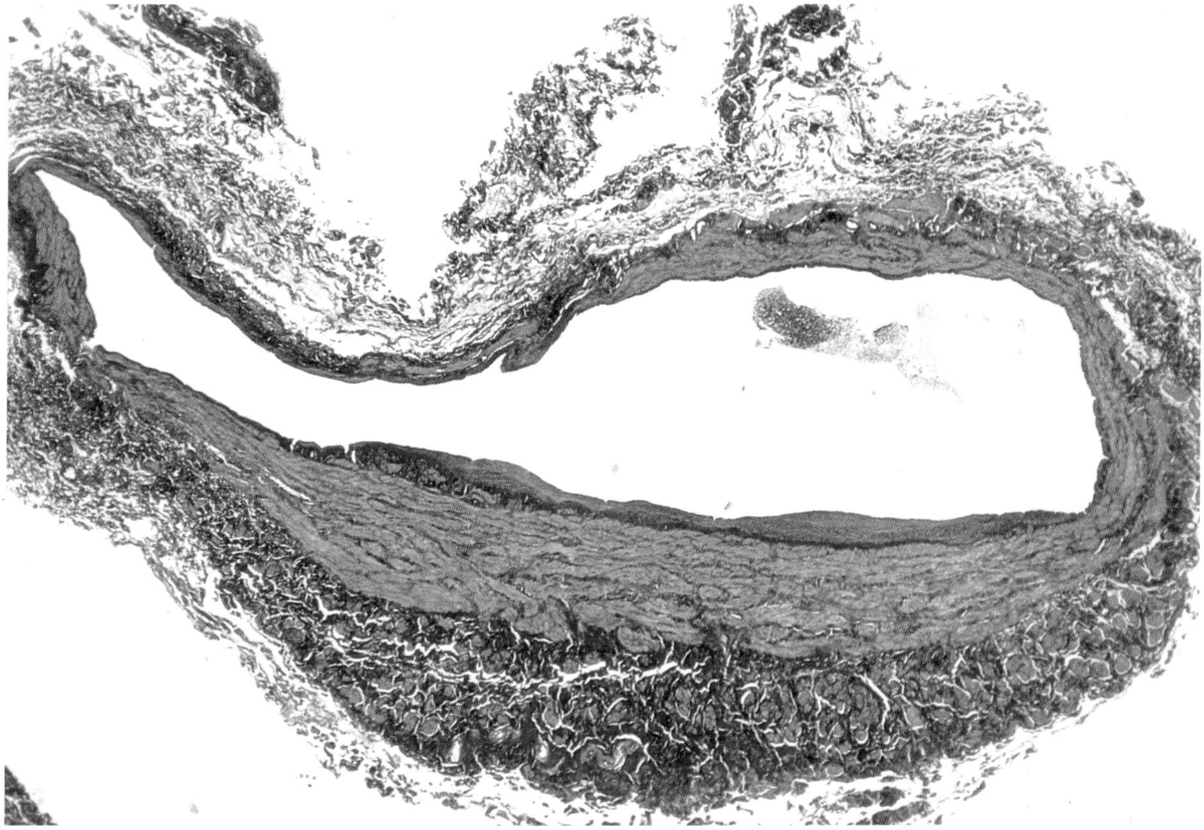

127

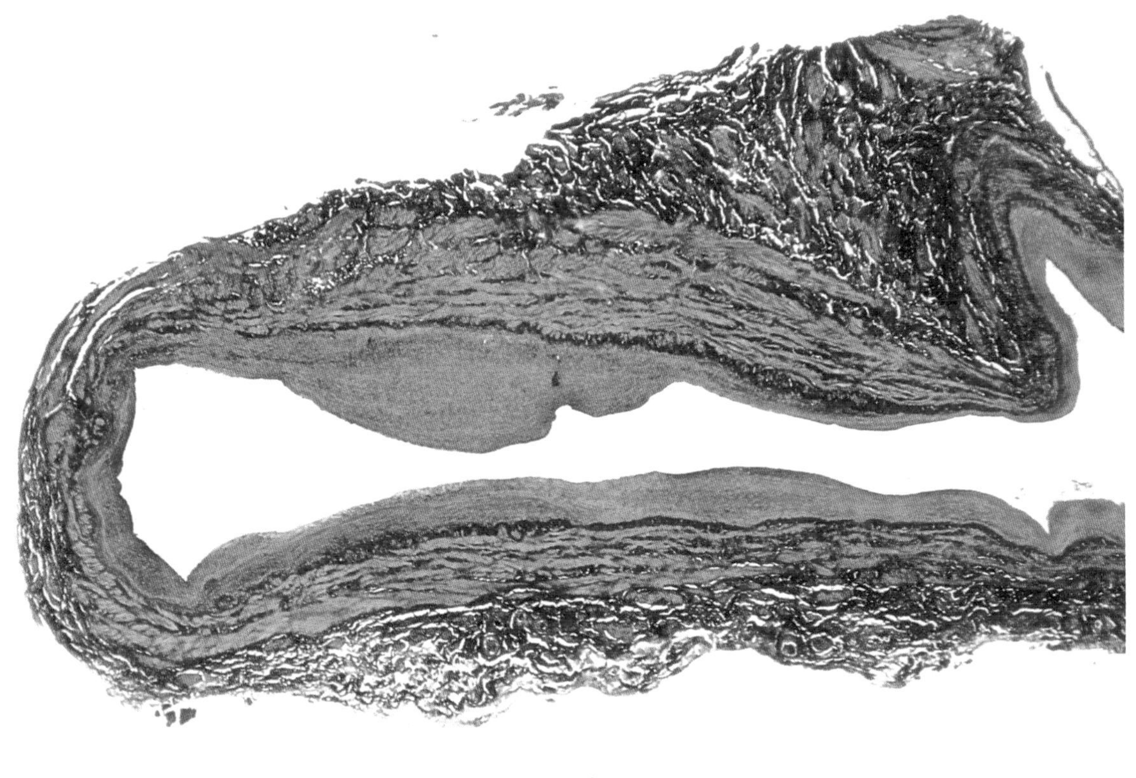

127: Moderate to marked varicosis with moderately severe phlebosclerosis: juxtaposition of hypertrophy/ hyperplasia and atrophy of the muscularis of the media with marked dilatation and outpouching of the lumen. Bands and cushions of marked intima fibrosis (fibrous endophlebosclerosis). Mild increase of collagen fibrils and elastic fibres in the muscularis of the media. Variable, overall moderate to marked fibrous-elastic-muscular widening of the adventitia (periphlebosclerosis).
Segment of the right long saphenous vein of a 46-year-old woman (E.-#4233/90). ElHvG. Magnif. 1.25 × objective.

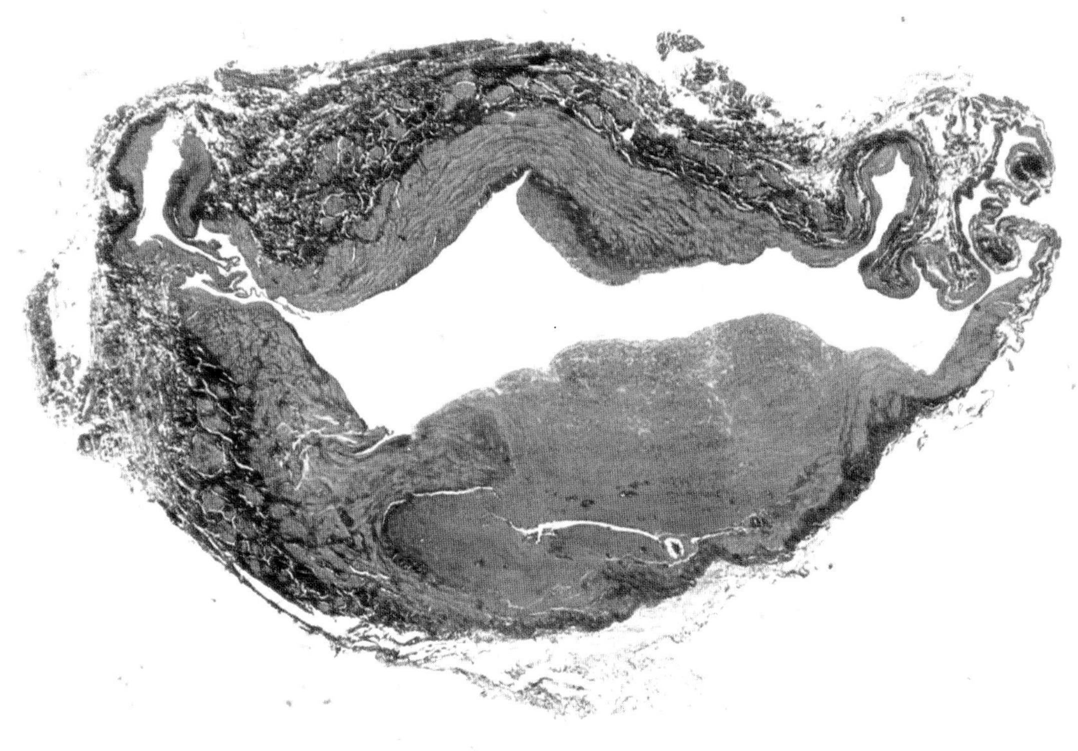

128: Moderate varicosis with destructive phlebosclerosis: partially thinned, partially widened muscularis of the media with mild increase of collagen and elastin. Small fibromuscular intima cushion (above) and replacement of the intima and a large portion of the media by moderately cellular, moderately vascularized fibrous connective tissue (below). Dilatation and outpouching of the lumen with thinning of the venous wall (on both sides). Marked fibrous-elastic-muscular widening of the adventitia (partial periphlebosclerosis, most pronounced in the left half of the figure). Partial sclerosis of the involved venous valves. Segment of the left long saphenous vein of a 46-year-old woman (E.-#8504/90). ElHvG. Magnif. 1.25 × objective.

129

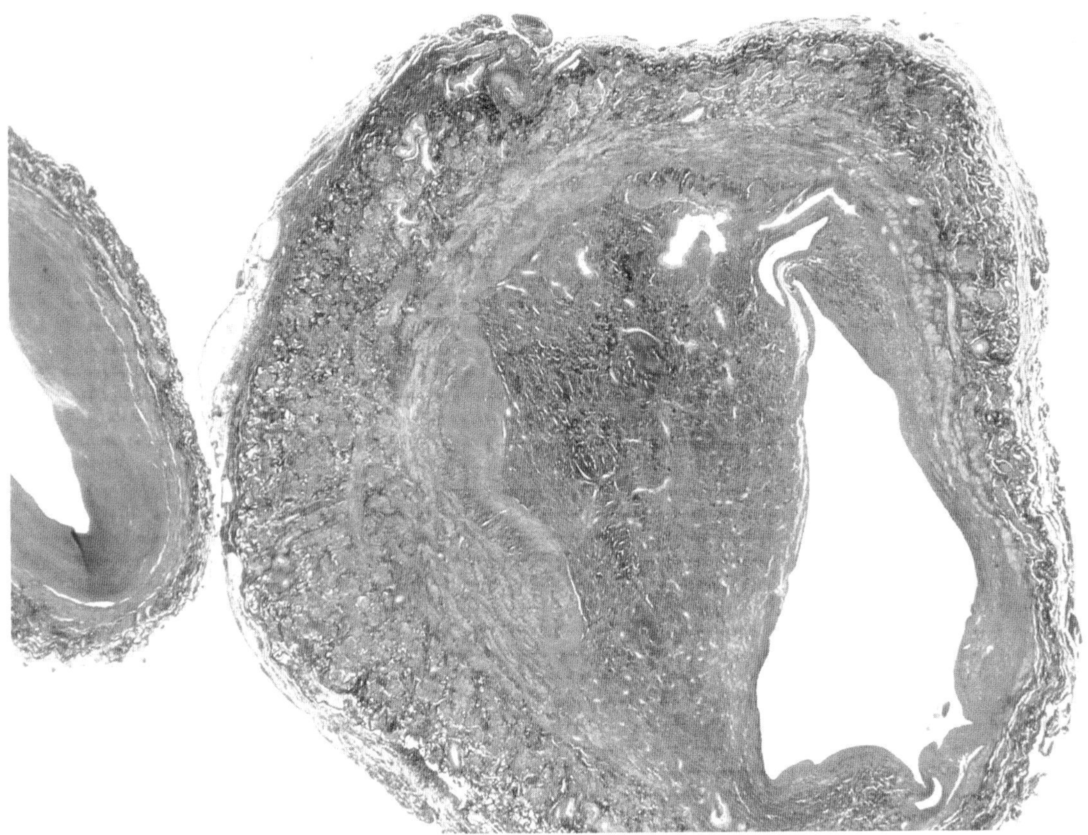

129: Recanalization of an older, organized thrombosis in a case of marked varicosis with phlebosclerosis. The muscularis of the media has a varying thickness and is criss-crossed by collagen fibrils. On the right side the lumen shows outpouchings. The intima shows a circular band-like fibrous thickening and is partially hyalinized; left above and left below, the intima has been partially destroyed and replaced by the organizing tissue, which has spread to the media (destructive sclerosis). The adventitia is thin on the right side of the figure but shows marked fibrous-elastic-muscular widening on the left (partial periphlebosclerosis). Segment of the right long saphenous vein of a 79-year-old woman (E.-#7006/90). ElHvG. Magnif. 1.25 × objective.

130

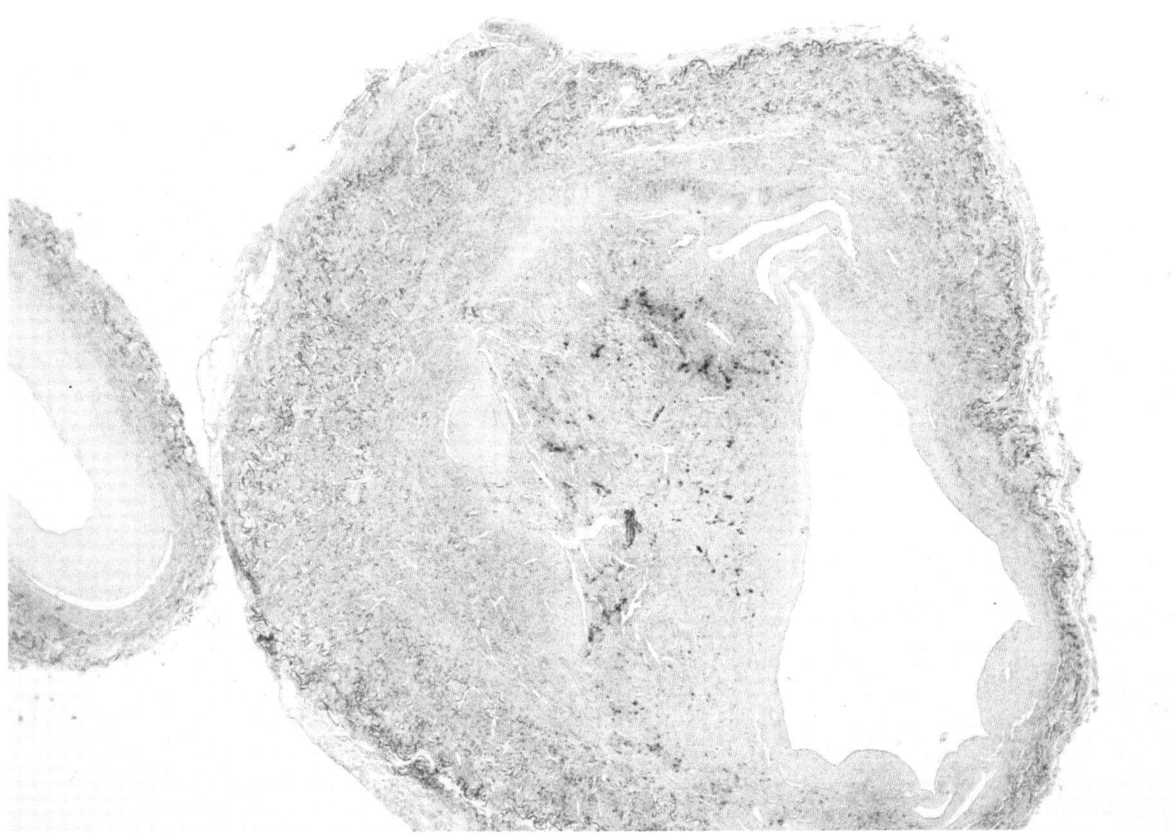

130: Same specimen. Close to capillaries in the organized old thrombus, numerous macrophages laden with haemosiderin can be seen, as well as stored haemosiderin outside cells. The iron pigment is stained blue. Berlin blue reaction.

131

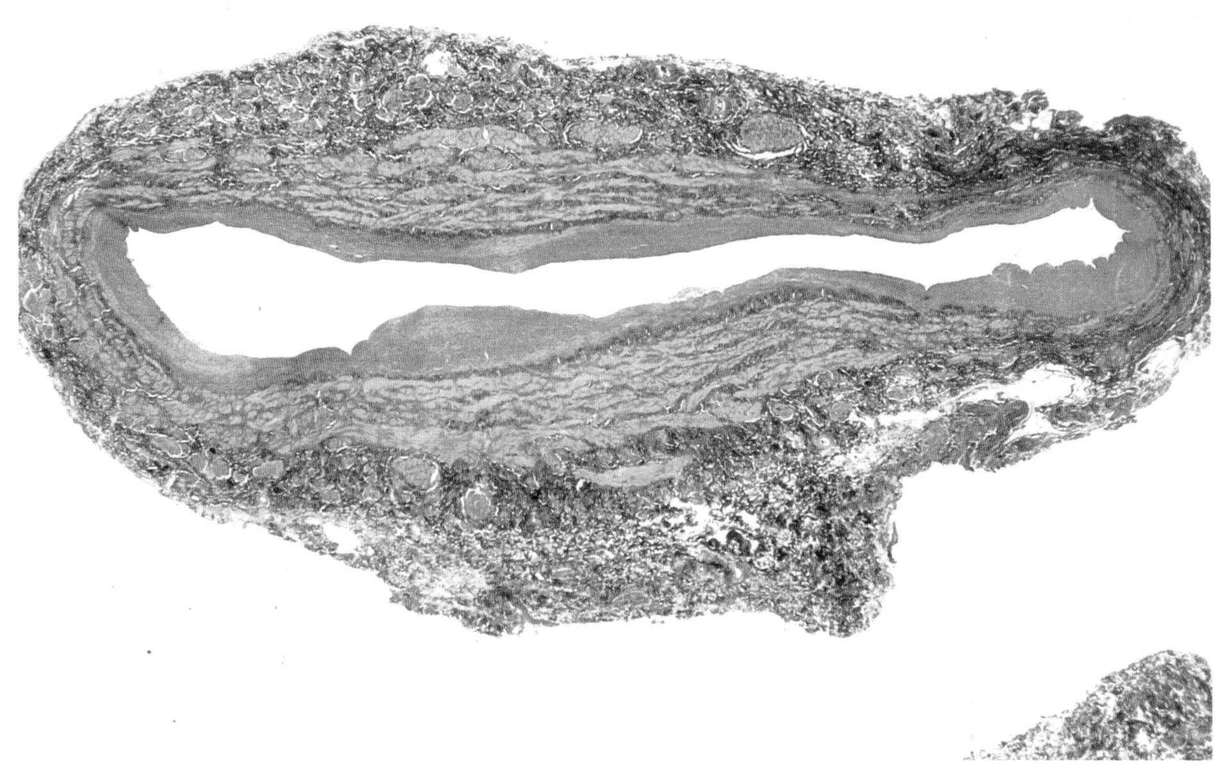

131: Moderate varicosis with moderate phlebosclerosis and a tiny platelet thrombus. The muscularis of the media shows varying width and is criss-crossed with collagen fibrils and a few elastic fibres. The lumen shows some outpouching. The intima shows circular, band-like fibrous thickening, in some places enlarged to cushions (endophlebosclerosis). The adventitia is partially mildly, partially markedly widened by collagen fibrils, elastic fibres and longitudinal smooth muscle fibres (partial periphlebosclerosis).
In the lower part of the venous wall, about the middle, the intima is covered by a tiny platelet thrombus. Segment of the right long saphenous vein of a 46-year-old woman. (E.-#4233/90). ElHvG. Magnif. 1.25 × objective.

132: Same specimen. The small platelet thrombus consists of thrombocytes and a few loose endothelial cells, some mononuclear cells, and a very few short fibrin strands. Magnif. 10 × objective.

133: Same specimen. Magnif. 25 × objective.

132

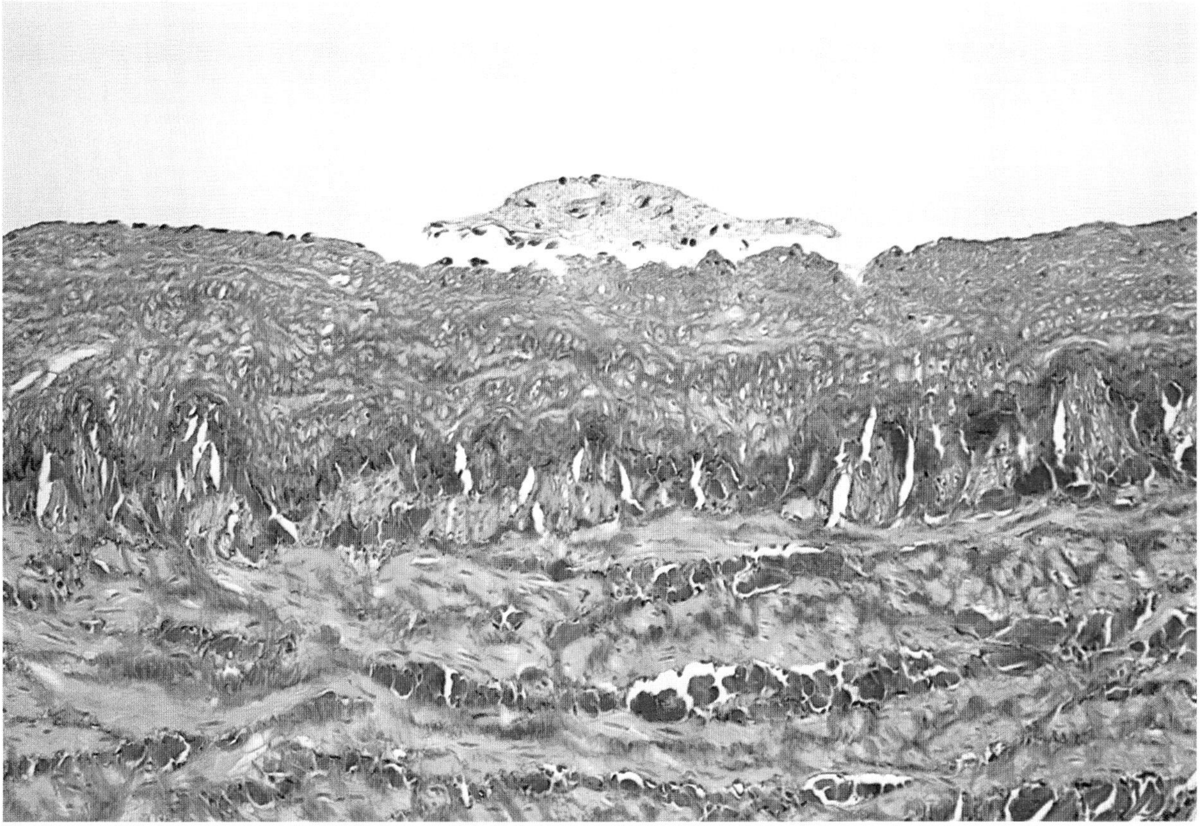

133

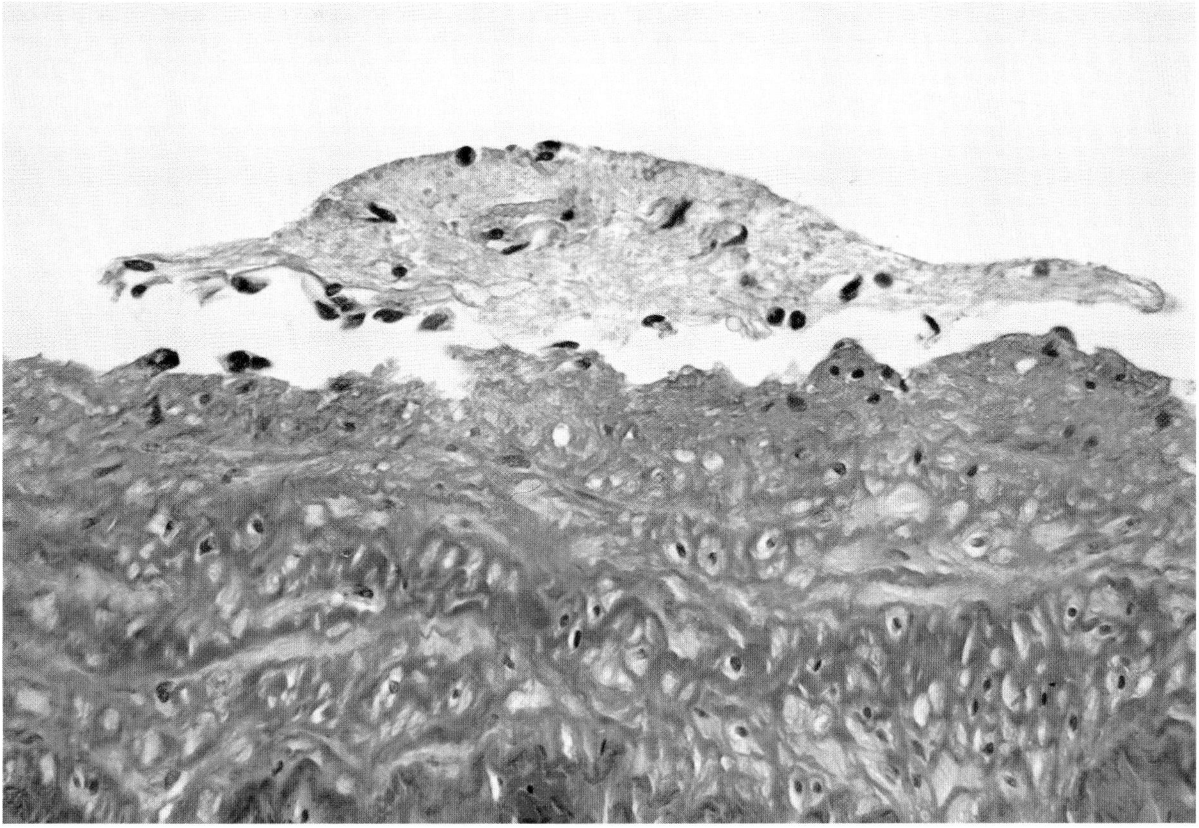

134

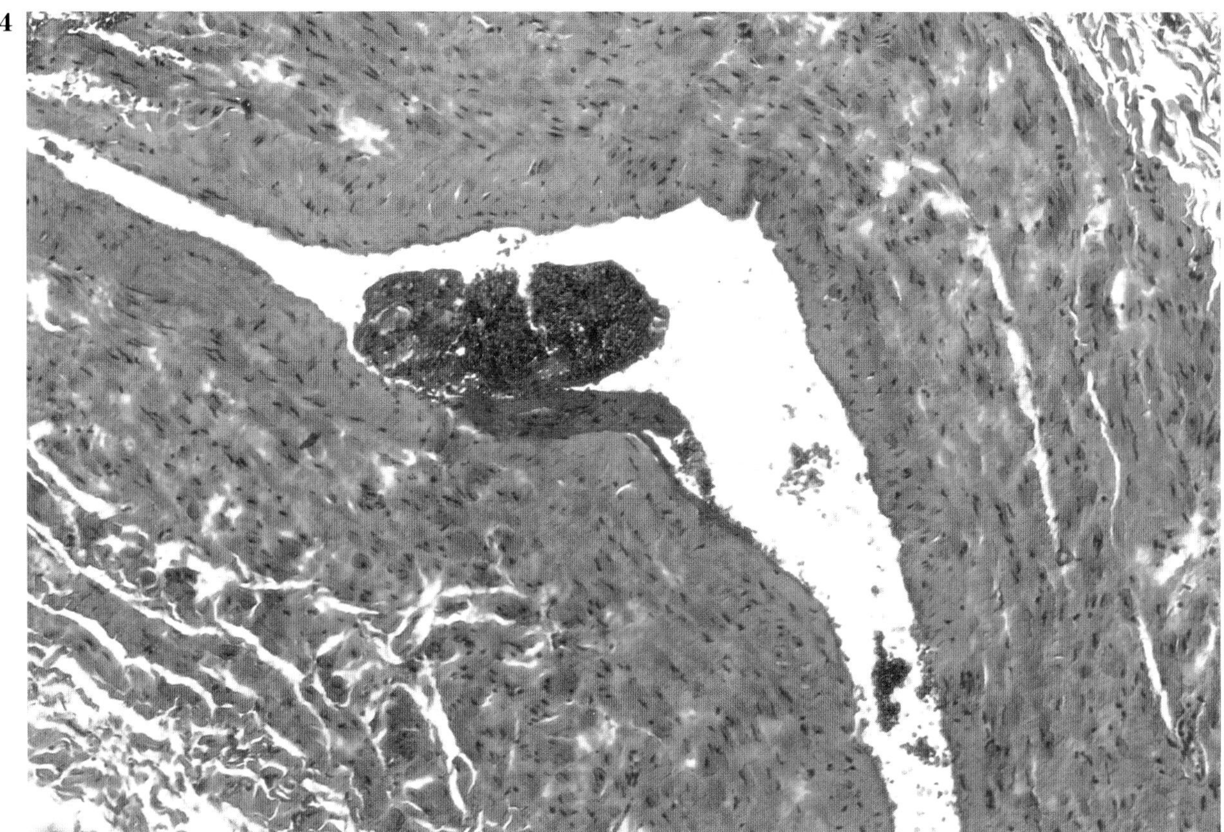

134: Small fresh precipitation thrombus which was built in layers. Segments of a vein wall with moderate varicosis; mild, in some areas cushion-like, fibromuscular endophlebosclerosis; mild fibromuscular periphlebosclerosis.
Right long saphenous vein of a 46-year-old woman. (E.-#6007/90). HE. Magnif. 6.3 × objective.

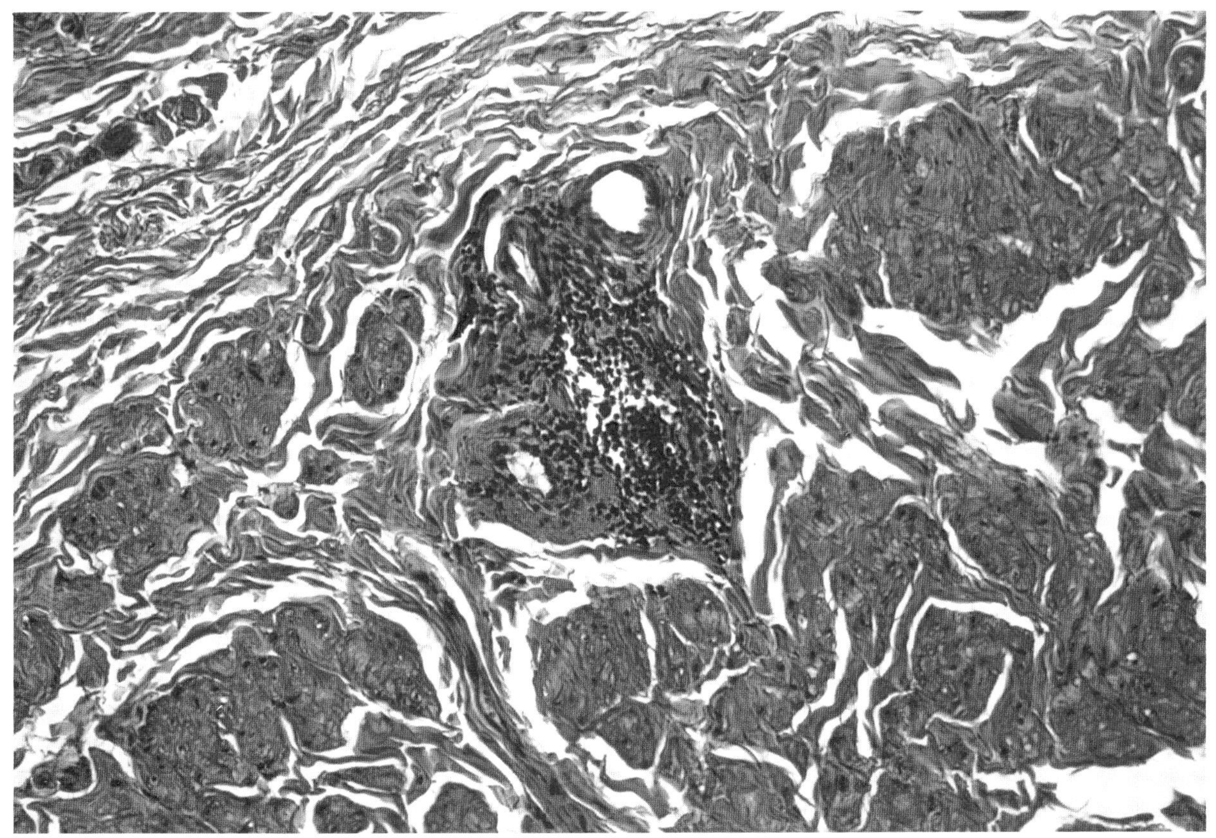

135

135: Small foci of intramural chronic phlebitis: small focus of mononuclear round cells between two vasa vasorum.
Segment of a venous wall with moderate varicosis, moderate cushion-like fibrous endophlebosclerosis, mild media fibrosis and more advanced fibrous-elastic-muscular periphlebosclerosis.
Segment of the right long saphenous vein of a 56-year-old woman. (E.-#4234/90). HE. Magnif. 10 × objective.

136

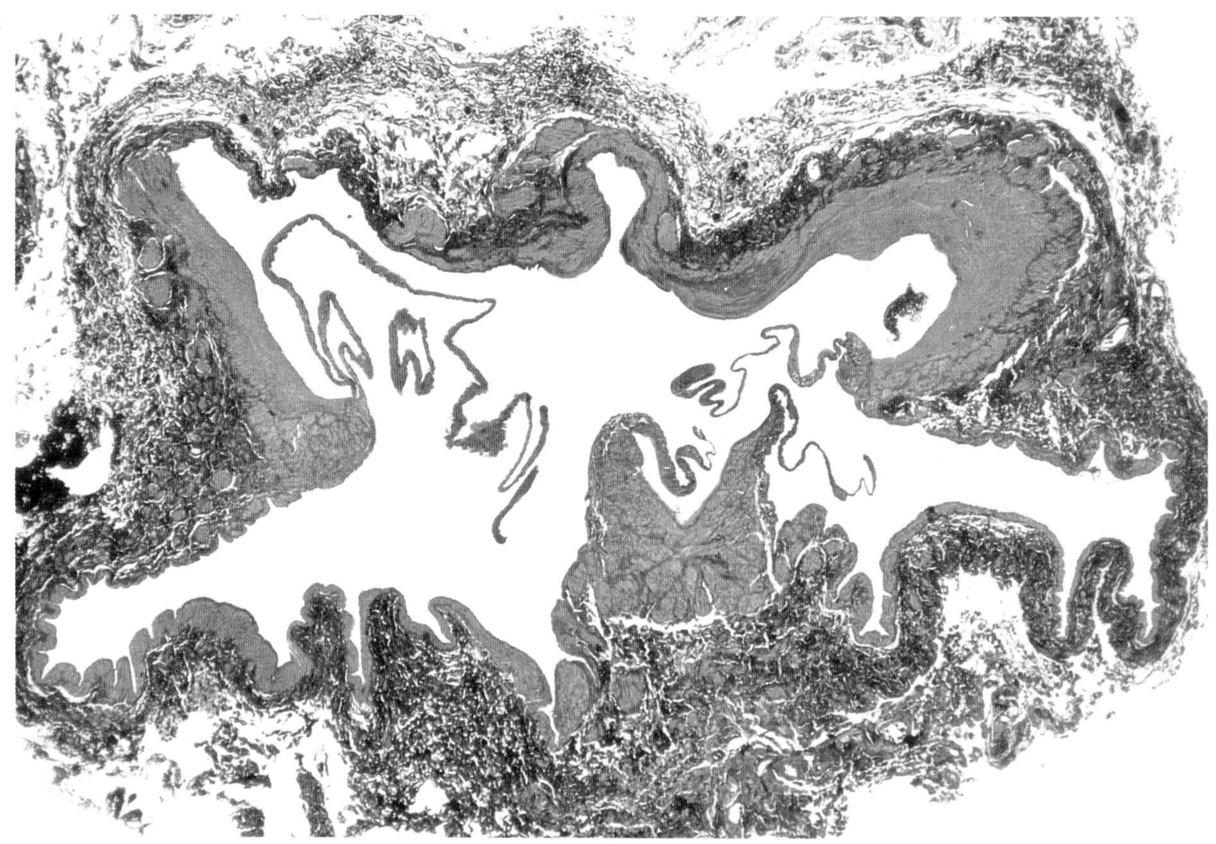

136: Mild partial venous valvular sclerosis at the entrance of two venous tributaries into the long saphenous vein. The valvular stroma is partially delicate, partially mildly widened by fibrous tissue.
Intermediate varicosis of the long saphenous vein with moderate endophlebosclerosis and more advanced varicosis of the tributaries. Varying degrees of fibroelastic periphlebosclerosis and only mild muscular periphlebosclerosis.
Segment of the right long saphenous vein with tributaries of a 41-year-old woman. (E.-#3616/90 I). ElHvG. Magnif. 1.25 × objective.

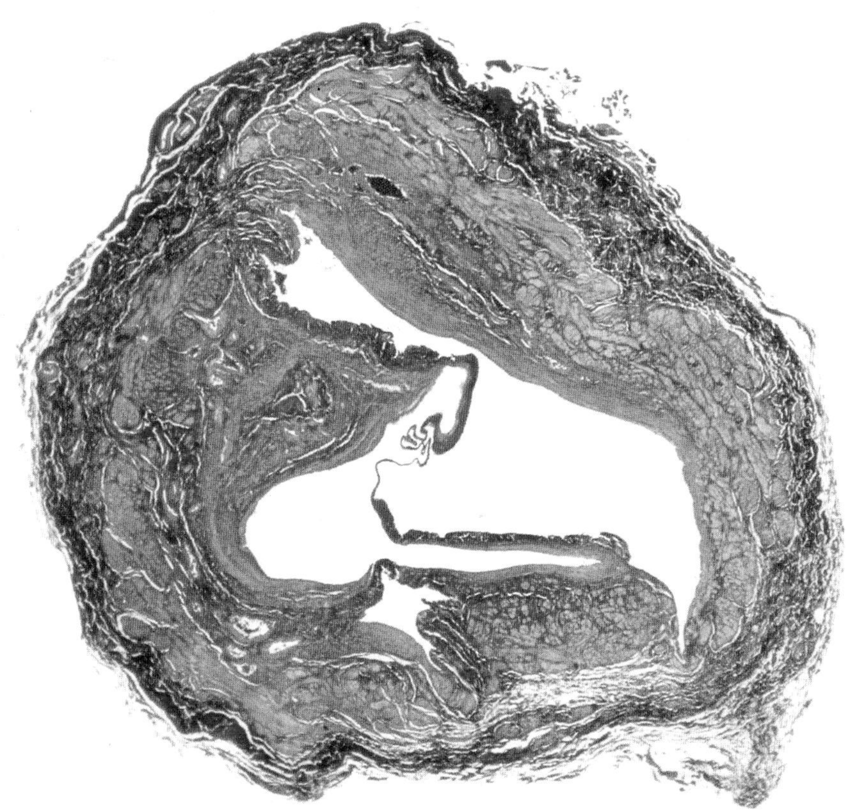

137: Intermediate partial venous valvular sclerosis at the entrance of a small tributary into the long saphenous vein. The valvular stroma is partially delicate, partially shows more marked fibrous thickening and sclerosis. Intermediate varicosis and phlebosclerosis.
Segment of the left long saphenous vein of a 43-year-old male. (E.-#7446/90). ElHvG. Magnif. 1.25 × objective.

138

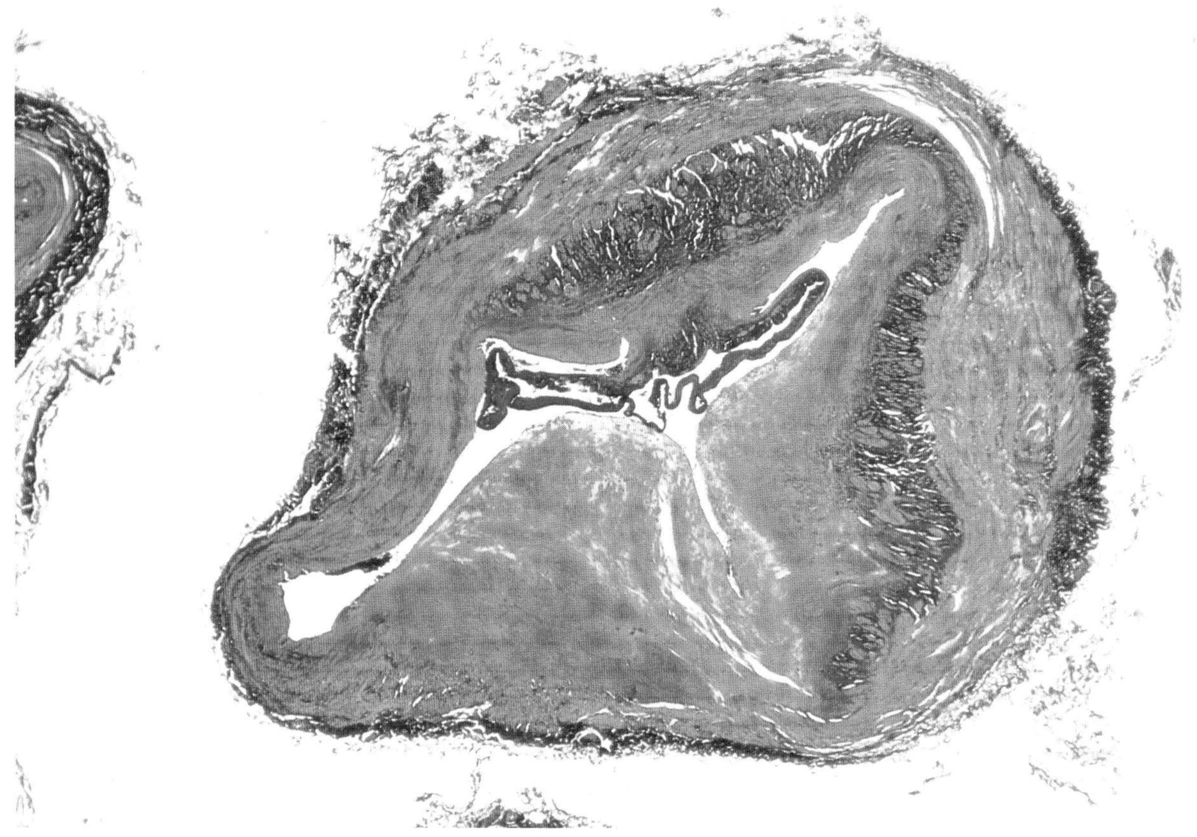

138: Marked valvular sclerosis at the entrance of a small vein into a tributary of the long saphenous vein. The valvular stroma shows moderate to marked fibrous thickening and sclerosis.
Intermediate varicosis with marked, partially destructive endophlebosclerosis of the tributary.
Right long saphenous vein with tributary of a 46-year-old woman. (E.-#6007/90). ElHvG. Magnif. 1.25 × objective.

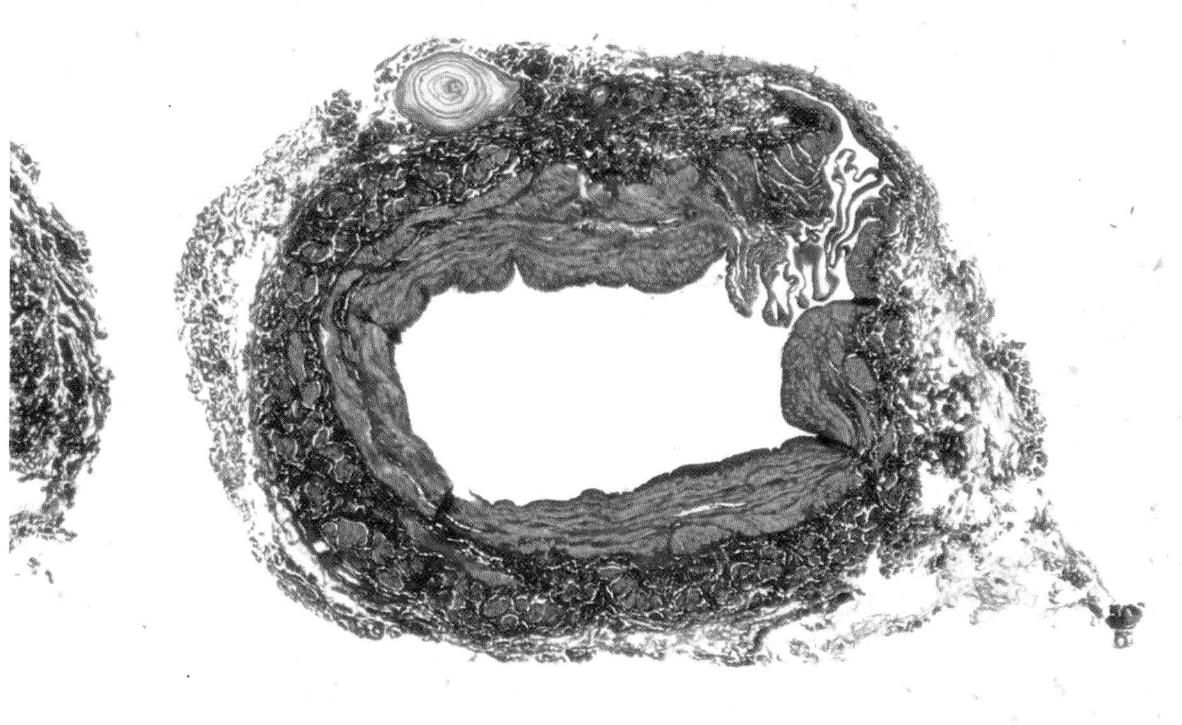

139: Small tactile corpuscle of the Vater-Pacini type in the adventitia of the tributary.
Mild varicosis. Mild to moderate valvular sclerosis. No true endophlebosclerosis. Moderate fibrous-elastic-muscular periphlebosclerosis.
Segment of a tributary of right long saphenous vein. 54-year-old woman. (E.-#7494/90). ElHvG. Magnif. 1.25 × objective.

Select bibliography

The following is a list of some basic sources of information in the English phlebology literature. It is not meant to be complete, but is intended as an introduction and orientation.

BROWSE, N. L., BURNAND, K. G., LEA, T. M.: Diseases of the Veins: Pathology, Diagnosis and Treatment, London, Edward Arnold, 1988.
A very complete textbook on the modern treatment of venous disorders.

GOLDMAN, M. P.: Sclerotherapy: Treatment of Varicose and Telangiectatic Leg Veins, St. Louis, Mosby-Year Book, 1991.
The first U.S. textbook on the modern treatment of superficial venous disorders, with the accent on practical sclerotherapy. The book also gives excellent reviews of the historical development of most treatment methods.

BERGAN, J. J. and GOLDMAN, M. P.: Varicose Veins and Telangiectasias: Diagnosis and Treatment, St. Louis, Quality Medical Publishing, 1993.
An anthology of chapters on different aspects of varicose vein treatment by a group of international authors.

DE GROOT, W. P.: Practical Phlebology, Sclerotherapy of Large Veins, J. Dermatol. Surg. Oncol. **17**, 589–595 (1991).
A clear description of the modern concept of the origin of reflux in varicose veins and its influence on the complementary roles of surgery and sclerotherapy in modern treatment, together with practical guidelines for sclerotherapy.

JOURNAL OF DERMATOLOGIC SURGERY AND ONCOLOGY, Elsevier, New York.
The official organ of the North American Society of Phlebology (together with three other societies). Every three months a section of this journal is devoted to papers on practical phlebology as well as research.

PHLEBOLOGY, Springer-Verlag, London.
The official organ of the Venous Forum of the Royal Society of Medicine (England) and the Societas Phlebologica Scandinavica. Second largest English-language phlebology journal. Appears four times per year. It tends to be somewhat more theoretical and surgically oriented than the Journal of Dermatologic Surgery and Oncology.

Index

A

Adaptation, morphological, 91
Adventitia, 91
Adventitial fibrosis, 93
Age-related fibrosis, 91
Age-related changes, 91
Anastomosis, arteriovenous, 82
Aneurysm, venous, 38, 93
Angiodysplasia, 82
Arteries, epifascial, 24
Artery, communicating, 27
-perforating, 22, 23
-anterior tibial, 25
Arterioles, 59
Atrophie blanche, 59, 74

B

Bandages, high stretch resistence, 77
Blow out, 47, 74
Branch varicosis, 28, 30, 38

C

Calf veins, incompetence, 45
Circulation disturbances, 91
Claudication symptoms, 79
Coagulation thrombosis, 94, 96
Collagen, 92
Collateral circulation, 51
Compression therapy, 77, 87
-stockings, 88
-bandages, 88
Contact eczema, 61
Connective tissue cells, 91
Corona phlebectatica paraplantaris, 41, 58

D

Deep veins, 31
-incompetence, 44, 45
Dependency syndrome, 30
Diabetes mellitus, 80, 81
Dodd perforator, 47
Doppler examination, 55
Dow's sign, 45
Duplex ultrasonography, 36, 68

E

Eczema, 61
Eczema craquelé, 61
Elastin, 92
Endophlebosclerosis, 93, 108
Erysipelas, 63, 89

F

Fascia, crural, 15
-dorsal, of foot, 15
-lata, 13
Fat collar, supramalleolar, 90
Feeder vein, 49
Femoro-popliteal incompetence, 42, 43
Fibres, elastic, 93
Fibrils, 91
Fibrosis, diffuse reticular, 93
Fibrosis, of inner layer, 93
Fistulas, 91
Flow phenomena, 48
Fossa ovalis, 13

G

Gaiter ulcer, 60
Gangrene, diabetic, 80
Giacomini's vein, 35

H

Haemodynamics, 93
History, phlebological, 10
Hyperpigmentation, 47, 59
Hyperplasia, 93
Hypertrophy, 93
Hypodermitis, 61

I

Intima, 94
-fibrosis, 93

K

Kinking, 42
Klippel-Trenaunay syndrome, 82

L

Leg swelling, 86
Leg veins, 91
-thrombosis, 72
Lentigo maligna melanoma, 78
Ligation and Division (of long saphenous vein), 41, 54, 88
Light Reflexion Rheography, 56
Lipoedema, 90
Lipoma, 48
Lymph nodes, 86
-oedema, 87
Lymphatic scintigraphy, 86

M

Macroangiopathy, 80
Malum perforans, 81
Media, circular, 91
-fibrosis, 93, 94
-longitudinal, 91
Medial malleolus, 26
Microangiopathy, 80, 81
Muscle fibres, 91
Muscle cells, smooth, 92
Myocytes, 91

N

Necrobiosis lipoidica, 78
Neuropathy, 81

O
Occlusion, thrombotic, 66
Oedema, 83, 85
-lymphatic, 85
-lymphatic, in malignancy, 87
Oedema, venous, 77

P
Pedal pulse, 79
Pelvic venous outflow pathways, 52
-thrombosis, 68, 75
-occlusion, 86
Perforator varicosis, 28, 47
-veins, 46
-incompetence, 75
Periphlebosclerosis, 93, 94, 100
Phlebitis, acute, 94
-intramural, chronic, 105
-chronic, with small foci, 94
Phlebosclerosis, 93
-destructive, 94, 95, 99
-fibromuscular, 93
-moderate, 98, 102
Phlegmasia cerulea dolens, 64
Photoplethysmography, 56
Pigmentation changes, 59
Pits, 85
Platelets, 96
-thrombi, 94
-thrombus, 102
Precipitation thrombosis, 94
-thrombus, 104
Pressure ulcer, 81

R
'Railroad tracking', 71
Ramus fibularis, 25
-musculocutaneous magnus, 26
Recurrent varicosis, 54
Reverse flow, 93

S
Saphenofemoral junction incompetence, 30, 41
Septum, anterior intermuscular, 25
Skin, pitting, 83
-nerves, 14
-changes, trophic, 58
Soft tissue trauma, 62
Spider veins, 49
Spontaneous De Palma operation, 51
Squamous cell carcinoma, 77
Stasis ulcers, 74
Stasis, venous, 75
Status, venous, 10
Stemmer's sign, 85

T
Tactile corpuscle, 109
Thrombophlebitis, 62, 94
Thrombosis, 94, 95
Thrombosis, of deep veins, 85, 86
Thrombus, 67
Truncal varicosis, 28, 29, 32, 39, 40, 41
Truncus tibiofibularis, 27

U
Ulcer, mixed, 78
-postphlebitic, 73
-stasis, 73
-varicose, 73
Ulceration, 73

V
Valsalva manoeuvre, 55
Valve destruction, 68
-incompetence, 43, 93
Varices, primary, 92
-secondary, 92
-suprapubic, 52
Varices, types, 28
Varicose veins, 92
Varicosis, primary, 30
-secondary, 30
Varicosis, 92, 93, 96
— mild, 96
— moderate, 98, 99, 102
— reticular, 28
Vein, posterior saphenous, 34
-posterior arch, 21
-long saphenous, 19, 21, 31, 47
-short saphenous, 20, 36
-incompetence, 44
-varicosis, 37
-perforating, 22, 23
Vein, posterior tibial, 66
Vein, superficial circumflex ilium, 12
-anterior crural, 39
-femoral, 67
Veins, superficial epigastric, 32
Veins, superficial, 14, 17, 18
-peripheral, 91
-central, 91
Venectasia, 58, 92
Venography, 33, 68
Venous flow, decreased, 68
Venous pressure, 93
-valves, 31, 94
-valvular sclerosis, 94, 106, 107
-thrombosis, deep, 68
-occlusion plethysmography, 68
-wall, 93
Venous stasis, 92
Venules, 93
Virchow's triad, 68
Vulvular varices, 53

W
Work-up of varicosis, 11